DR. ROBERT H. GOLDSTEIN

Real Self Care For Men

The Essential Guide To Physical And Mental Self-Care For Men

Contents

Introduction

Taking care of yourself encompasses a broad spectrum of activities, ranging from familiar routines like indulging in a lengthy shower or hitting the gym to more unconventional acts such as disconnecting from your phone, foregoing caffeine, and experimenting with meditation. In the digital era, social media showcases diverse practices labeled as self-care, reflecting its evolution into a cultural phenomenon. At its essence, self-care involves engaging in activities that bring about a sense of well-being and prioritizing personal wellness. It goes beyond merely feeling good; self-care contributes to improved health, enhanced stress management, longevity, and even a more refined physical appearance.

While societal norms have often framed self-care as a predominantly female practice, this perception is debunked in "Real Self-Care for Men." This book challenges stereotypes, emphasizing that self-care knows no gender, race, class, or sexual orientation. Acknowledging that men, in particular, tend to neglect self-care, the book aims to demystify and simplify the concept. Self-care doesn't demand an exhaustive time commitment; it comprises simple, accessible actions that yield immediate benefits.

"Real Self-Care for Men" provides a versatile array of self-care practices, catering to both novices and those seeking fresh approaches. From basic routines like regular moisturizing to more unconventional choices like getting a tattoo, the book encourages readers to view these acts as integral to self-care. It underscores the significance of personal grooming not only as a necessity but as a tangible expression of care for one's body, instigating a positive ripple effect on both inner and outer well-being.

The book introduces surprising facets of self-care that may initially raise eyebrows. Can blow-drying your hair be considered self-care? Absolutely. Do crystals have the power to influence your well-being? Indeed, they do. Does having a houseplant impact your mood? Scientifically proven, it does. The underlying message is clear: self-care is a personal journey, and the diverse practices explored in the book aim to inspire and broaden perspectives.

Ultimately, "Real Self-Care for Men" emphasizes that no one is coercing readers into adopting these practices. Rather, it invites them to explore the transformative potential of self-care, assuring that the positive impact can be both surprising and profound. The invitation is extended to open minds, encouraging individuals to embark on a journey of self-care that aligns with their unique preferences and needs.

Part 1 : The Mind

You may have noticed on social media that many self-care practices emphasize relaxing the body and reducing stress and anxiety. This focus stems from the tangible impact stress and anxiety can have on both the body and mind. However, there's a tendency to concentrate on external aspects, overlooking internal well-being, particularly mental health. This section includes conventional practices like meditation for calmness and surprising insights such as extending your self-care routine beyond home as a mental practice. Considering that anxiety often arises from external sources, why limit self-care to home? Equipping yourself with tools to manage stress in various life situations, especially when away from home, is crucial. Ultimately, prioritizing mental health is vital for everyone, and self-care is a key tool for improvement. Nevertheless, it's essential to recognize that self-care is just one aspect; if you suspect a serious mental health issue, seeking professional help is crucial. For those times when you feel overwhelmed, here are some solutions.

Meditation

When the term "meditation" comes up, the mental image often involves a tranquil Buddhist monk atop a mountain, seemingly untouched by the outside world. This individual is envisioned as having achieved enlightenment after spending days or even years in profound meditation. However, the reality of meditation is far simpler than relocating to a Himalayan monastery. Meditation is accessible to everyone, and a surprising number of people incorporate it into their lives. Contrary to the stereotypical image of someone chanting "om" at home on a Friday night, meditation can be uncomplicated, brief, and practiced anywhere. Consider your mind as a muscle, and meditation as the exercise that strengthens it, without necessarily focusing on the brain itself.

Meditation, in simple terms, involves clearing your mind by directing your awareness and training your focus on a single thing to eliminate other distractions. The objective is to attain a sustained state of calm. Despite its apparent simplicity, beginners often find meditation challenging, grappling with the difficulty of clearing their minds and avoiding entanglement in thoughts. This frustration might lead them to perceive meditation as too difficult. However, many instructors emphasize that meditation is inherently challenging for everyone, hence why it's referred to as a practice. Achieving the ability to completely clear your mind requires skill and experience, and even individuals with years of meditation may still find it elusive. Meditating is about the journey and experience; successful meditation is an ongoing process, not a fixed destination.

Why Engage in Meditation?

Meditation, an age-old practice spanning various cultures, has been employed for centuries. Recent scientific research reveals tangible impacts on both the body and mind. It is documented to reduce blood pressure, slow heart rate, and enhance overall blood circulation. Many meditation techniques emphasize breath work, contributing to a physical slowdown of breathing and increased oxygen circulation in the bloodstream.

In terms of mental well-being, meditation has proven to diminish anxiety, alleviate stress, uplift mood, and decrease cortisol levels in the brain. Studies indicate that individuals with regular meditation practices continue to experience these benefits even outside their meditation sessions. Practitioners find improved long-term management of anxiety and stress as a result of consistent meditation.

Varieties of Meditation

Meditation serves as a mental exercise, akin to physical workouts, and, similar to fitness routines, there exists a multitude of approaches. No single method fits everyone. Here are some prevalent styles of meditation.

Mindfulness

Among the various meditation styles, mindfulness stands out as one of the most popular. Rooted in the acceptance that completely clearing your mind might be challenging, mindfulness meditation encourages acknowledging thoughts without judgment, letting them pass through your mind. Typically, it involves focusing on a specific element, such as your breath, to redirect attention away from thoughts.

Transcendental

Widely recognized globally and extensively studied scientifically, Transcendental Meditation is structured and favored by celebrities like the Beatles, David Lynch, Jerry Seinfeld, and Ellen DeGeneres. It entails concentrating on a mantra, a repeated word or phrase to focus thoughts. Learning Transcendental Meditation often requires seeking guidance from an accredited teacher.

Mantra

Utilizing a repeated word or phrase, known as a mantra, mantra meditation aims to clear the mind by directing focus to these chosen words. This type can be beneficial for those who find focusing on breath challenging or sitting with their thoughts intimidating, offering a tangible activity.

Guided

With the surge in meditation's popularity, guided meditation through apps and classes has become prevalent. In this style, a voice or teacher leads you through the meditation, guiding visualization or instructing breath work and mindfulness. Guided meditation is particularly suitable for beginners who may struggle with sitting in silence for an extended duration.

Movement

Addressing the challenge some face with extended sitting, movement meditation allows individuals to engage in physical activities like yoga, walking, or household chores. The goal is not to elevate heart rate but to let the body go on autopilot, enabling the mind to focus inward.

How to Begin Meditating

Initiating a meditation practice, regardless of the chosen style, can be a significant challenge for beginners. Many individuals feel intimidated by the prospect of meditation, thinking they must endure prolonged periods of silence to succeed. It's essential to recognize that meditation is a process, not about achieving perfection from the outset. Be kind to yourself and accept discomfort; there is no concept of failure in meditation. To commence, follow these straightforward steps:

1. Find a comfortable position, whether sitting in a chair, on a meditation cushion, or lying down. Aim for a position that allows you to stay comfortable for around 20 minutes without being so comfortable that you risk falling asleep.

1. Close your eyes; if keeping them closed is challenging, consider using an eye mask to minimize distractions.

1. If you're new to meditation, allow your breath to flow naturally and deeply without attempting to control it.

1. Focus on the sensations of your breath within your body. Observe the air entering your nostrils or mouth, feel your lungs filling up, and notice your rib cage expanding. Keep your attention on your breath, gently bringing it back when your mind inevitably wanders.

1. Begin with short sessions, around 3–5 minutes. Practice daily, gradually extending the duration as you become more experienced. Aim to reach 15–20 minutes for each meditation session over time.

There's a Solution in the Digital Era

Thanks to modern advancements, initiating a meditation routine has become incredibly convenient. Numerous smartphone applications cater to various meditation styles, allowing you to explore, monitor your progress, and unwind swiftly on the go or during work hours. Many of these apps feature guided meditations, particularly beneficial for beginners. Simply plug in your headphones and meditate for a few minutes wherever you find yourself. Some apps even offer specialized meditations for specific objectives such as sleep, focus, stress relief, and happiness. While the meditations may vary subtly, the overarching aim remains consistent: simplifying and making meditation accessible.

Acupuncture

To those unfamiliar, acupuncture may appear mystical, with images of individuals lying on beds adorned with needles. How could such a practice be beneficial? In reality, acupuncture is an age-old remedy deeply rooted in Chinese medicine, and scientific evidence supports its efficacy in addressing both physical and mental conditions.

Understanding acupuncture requires delving into traditional Chinese medicine's perspective on the body. Envision the body as a roadmap, with various channels known as meridians traversing it. These meridians serve as energy pathways—some substantial, akin to highways, while others are smaller, resembling side streets or paths. Together, they facilitate the smooth flow of energy throughout the body. When unobstructed, energy reaches its intended destinations, maintaining overall balance. However, blockages, akin to traffic jams, can disrupt this flow, causing pain and various other issues in Chinese medicine.

Acupuncture emerges as a solution to clear these blockages. According to traditional Chinese medicine, specific points along the intricate meridian network, when stimulated, can open up pathways, allowing energy to circulate freely. Acupuncture, involving the insertion of tiny stainless steel needles superficially into the skin, serves as a method to activate these pressure points.

Benefits of Acupuncture

Typically, discussions about acupuncture tend to focus on its effectiveness in addressing physical ailments. It has proven to be a valuable tool in relieving various types of pain, including muscle and joint issues, as well as chronic inflammation within the body. Acupuncture is utilized for conditions such as chronic heart problems, respiratory issues, gastrointestinal disorders, and fatigue. Additionally, it can target superficial concerns like skin and hair problems by enhancing blood flow to the surface.

Less commonly emphasized is acupuncture's capacity to address non-physical ailments. Research indicates that acupuncture can contribute to the alleviation of anxiety, depression, fear, and even addiction. A widely recognized application of acupuncture is in smoking cessation. Furthermore, it has demonstrated effectiveness in treating more severe anxiety disorders like post-traumatic stress disorder (PTSD) and social anxiety disorder.

Selecting an Acupuncturist

Acupuncture is a highly specialized field requiring extensive study, often spanning years or even decades. Choosing an acupuncturist demands careful consideration. While some practitioners may hold medical degrees, this should not be the sole criterion. Look for specific certifications in acupuncture and Chinese medicine. Exploring terms like "homeopath" or "naturopath" could also be beneficial, as these holistic doctors may possess training in acupuncture, herbalism, and other alternative medical practices.

Conduct thorough research. Despite its seemingly straight-forward nature, acupuncture requires precision, and complications may arise if not performed correctly or in an unclean environment. Utilize online review platforms, scrutinizing each review, with particular attention to the average rating rather than extreme opinions. Seeking recommendations from your primary doctor is also advisable, as many medical professionals now endorse acupuncture as a complementary treatment.

Ultimately, trust your instincts. Your initial choice is not binding; if you don't resonate with a practitioner after the first appointment, consider exploring other providers until you find a suitable match.

Your Inaugural Acupuncture Session

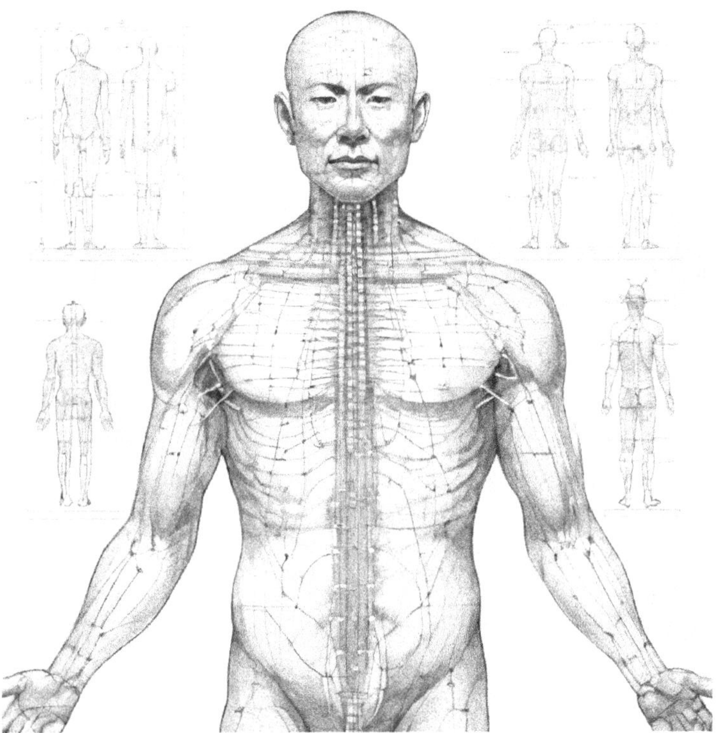

Approach your first acupuncture appointment much like any other visit to a medical professional, given that acupuncture is a specialized medical discipline. Here's what you can anticipate:

1. Consultation: The initial session will commence with a thorough discussion of the ailments you aim to address through acupuncture. Be transparent, treating it akin to a checkup with your regular doctor. Expect inquiries about your diet, lifestyle, stress levels, and past and present medical conditions.

2. Evaluation: Your practitioner will likely conduct various

assessments, including pulse-taking, examining your tongue and mouth, and exploring areas for pain or inflammation. Unconventional methods might involve inspecting your face's color, scrutinizing your feet, or employing tools like crystals or a pendulum to assess energy flow.

3. Treatment Plan: The acupuncturist will outline their course of action, specifying which body areas they will target with needles. It's important to note that acupuncture points may be distant from the site of physical pain. Relax, as understanding this complex system may take time. If clothing removal is necessary, the practitioner will inform you.

4. Needle Insertion: After lying back on a table, the practitioner will gently insert small needles into your skin. The process is superficial, and you may not feel anything. If you do, the acupuncturist will guide you through it.

5. Relaxation Period: Once the needles are in place, you'll be asked to relax for about 20 minutes as they take effect. The practitioner might create a soothing environment with dim lights and calming music. If you drift off to sleep, it's normal.

6. Needle Removal: After the session concludes, the acupuncturist will remove the needles. Depending on your condition, they may leave small tacks (seeds) on specific points to sustain energy flow post-session.

7. Post-Session Feelings: Post-acupuncture, some people feel relaxed, while others experience heightened energy levels. Sensations depend on the focus of the session and the ailment

being treated.

Time Management

The universal experience of feeling overwhelmed by too many tasks and too little time is something everyone can relate to. Uttering the phrase "there's not enough time in the day" is a common refrain. Many individuals, especially men, find that work is a significant source of anxiety due to the sheer volume of tasks and limited time available.

Unfortunately, it's not possible to create more time, but the silver lining is that you can develop skills to utilize your time more effectively. Time management emerges as a crucial skill, not only for enhanced productivity but also for reducing stress and anxiety. Essentially, time management is a form of self-care.

In essence, the more efficiently you manage your time, the less stress you'll experience. Beyond that, effective time management provides you with the opportunity to dedicate more time to self-care. If you find yourself thinking that activities like taking a bath or getting a full eight hours of sleep are unattainable, consider time management as your initial step toward prioritizing self-care.

How Effective Time Management Relieves Anxiety

Individuals lacking proficiency in time management often experience higher levels of anxiety, a sentiment amplified by the overwhelming daily task of "getting it all done" in today's hectic world. The indirect manner in which efficient time management aids in alleviating anxiety and stress is noteworthy. Feeling burdened by an insurmountable workload contributes to anxiety and may lead to procrastination, further intensifying feelings of guilt for unfinished tasks. Additionally, excessive responsibilities may prompt individuals to sacrifice sleep, detrimentally impacting physical and mental health (refer to Part 2 for further insights).

Addressing anxiety through time management doesn't necessitate completing the entire to-do list daily, but rather striving to do one's best. It also involves granting oneself the flexibility to adapt. Excessive rigidity can impede effective time management. As with many aspects of life, achieving balance is crucial, and finding the right equilibrium tailored to individual needs can significantly reduce stress levels.

Effective Time Management Strategies

Not every time management technique suits everyone, so it's advisable to experiment and find what works best for you. Here are some helpful starting points:

- Prep a To-Do List in Advance: Each evening, create a realistic list of tasks for the following day. Prioritize, placing essential tasks higher and less crucial ones lower. Starting the day with a plan can prevent feeling overwhelmed. Uncompleted tasks can be moved to the next day's list.

- Utilize a Calendar: Writing down appointments and deadlines in a calendar enhances memory. Include significant events and smaller goals to consolidate personal and work schedules. Employing a single calendar for both aspects of life streamlines organization.

- Establish Habits: Consistency is key for daily routines such as taking vitamins or creating a to-do list. Forming a habit may take approximately two months of regular practice. Tailor your habits to your goals and execute them daily for optimal effectiveness.

- Avoid Multitasking: While multitasking is often praised in the workplace, it can hinder time management. Concentrate on one task at a time to increase efficiency and minimize distractions, such as turning off the TV or using noise-canceling headphones.

- Embrace Time Blocking: Schedule dedicated blocks of

time for focused, single-tasking efforts. Ensure realistic time allocations, especially for more time-consuming tasks. Break larger tasks into manageable blocks, incorporating breaks or smaller tasks between them.

- Incorporate Short Breaks: Integrate short breaks, around 15 minutes, into your schedule, especially during longer tasks. Use this time to refresh by moving around, perhaps grabbing a drink, to maintain productivity without succumbing to procrastination.

- Allow Flexibility: Acknowledge that unexpected events will occur. When urgent tasks arise, reevaluate your to-do list and reprioritize accordingly. Adjust task priorities throughout the day, but ensure changes result from genuine requirements, not procrastination.

- Learn to Decline: Taking on excessive work often leads to heightened stress. Assess new tasks against your existing workload, and if adding them is unrealistic without sacrificing something else, consider declining. Learning to say no can positively impact stress levels.

- Prioritize Self-Care: In a world where external commitments dominate, ensure your schedule includes time for personal well-being. Whether scheduling a favorite workout or allowing time for a skincare routine, prioritizing self-care contributes to overall stress reduction.

On the move

Conversations on self-care often fall short by emphasizing activities confined to home, but considering our daily routines, we spend the majority of our time elsewhere. Whether at the office, commuting, or traveling, our presence at home is relatively limited compared to our on-the-go lifestyle. Consequently, constructing a self-care routine applicable anywhere becomes paramount.

A versatile self-care toolbox is essential, given that anxiety and stress stem from daily encounters in various environments—be it demanding work situations, traffic, or crowded stores. The cumulative effect of these experiences can become overwhelming. Relying solely on home-based practices, like taking a bath, may not be practical in the midst of a hectic day. Therefore, adapting your self-care routine to accommodate different locations is crucial.

Key components of self-care, such as self-check-ins and calming techniques, remain relevant regardless of your location. Simple practices like controlled breathing or using headphones for a meditation app can be effective in managing stress and anxiety, providing accessible solutions for moments of tension wherever you find yourself.

Significance

While the majority of this book delves into the ways self-care promotes relaxation, it's crucial to recognize that many individuals experience heightened anxiety when navigating the external world. Whether grappling with road rage, anxiety during flights, or discomfort in crowded spaces, self-care proves beneficial in addressing these challenges. A well-established self-care routine proves valuable wherever you are, particularly in navigating stressful situations that may not always unfold within the familiar confines of home.

Establishing a Mobile Self-Care Routine

Crucially, for any self-care routine, proactive planning is key. Whether embarking on a daily commute or preparing for an extended trip, consider the self-care methods you find beneficial at home and envision how they can be adapted to different environments. While it might not always be as straightforward as including a sheet mask in your carry-on, proactive planning ensures you have at least one self-care tool readily available for use whenever the need arises.

While Driving

Spending significant time in your car is a common reality, whether commuting or handling daily tasks. Transforming your car into a haven for self-care can greatly assist in stress management. Consider these practices:

1. Avoid work calls: Designate your car as a haven, free from work pressures. Refrain from taking work calls while driving, saving them for when you've completed your journey.

2. Silence your phone: Prevent anxiety and maintain focus on the road by switching your phone to silent mode, avoiding distractions from constant notifications.

3. Opt for podcasts: Instead of potentially lulling yourself to sleep with soothing music, choose podcasts. The conversational tone can be equally calming.

4. Engage in breathing exercises: While meditation isn't advised while driving, practicing controlled breathing can help manage stress, particularly in challenging situations like traffic jams or bouts of road rage.

5. Harness aromatherapy: Utilize aromatherapy in your car by incorporating a diffuser with natural essential oils like lavender. This can contribute to maintaining a calm and relaxed state during your journey.

At the Workplace

Given that many individuals dedicate a minimum of 40 hours per week to their jobs, and often more, incorporating self-care practices into the office routine can enhance the overall experience and aid in stress management. Consider the following strategies:

1. Take breaks from your desk: Regularly stepping away from

your desk, perhaps every hour, can promote blood circulation and sustain your energy levels throughout the day.

2. Organize your workspace: Maintaining a clutter-free desk is not just about tidiness; it can also contribute to reducing anxiety and creating a more focused work environment.

3. Introduce greenery: While outdoor breaks might be limited during the workday, having a plant on your desk can positively impact your mood and bring a touch of nature indoors.

4. Infuse pleasant scents: Lighting candles might not be feasible in an office setting, but using a small diffuser with essential oils can have a positive influence on your mood without causing disruptions.

5. Highlight your strengths: Amidst the workplace stress, focusing on your strengths and accomplishments can serve as a powerful reminder of your capabilities. Consider keeping a list at your desk to review during challenging moments.

6. Practice breathing exercises: If using a meditation app with headphones isn't feasible, a simple one-minute deep breathing exercise can effectively alleviate anxiety, providing a quick and discreet method for relaxation.

During Air Travel

Many individuals may identify themselves as apprehensive fliers, and even for those who don't, extended flights can induce stress due to various factors like cramped spaces, disturbances, and unfamiliar odors. Employing self-care strategies can help you navigate any flight smoothly.

1. Stretch periodically: Particularly on extended flights, taking short walks around the cabin is crucial for maintaining good blood circulation. You need not perform vigorous exercises but moving a bit can enhance circulation.

2. Utilize noise-canceling headphones: These can serve to muffle disruptive sounds, such as a crying baby nearby, allowing you to enjoy your meditation app undisturbed.

3. Pack nutritious snacks: Given the general dissatisfaction with airplane food, bringing your own healthy snacks can prevent that post-flight feeling of discomfort.

4. Prioritize skincare: The recycled air in planes can quickly dehydrate your skin. Packing essentials like cleansing wipes, moisturizer, and face mist can help keep your skin feeling refreshed, with bonus points for including a sheet mask.

5. In-flight massage: Especially on lengthy flights, using small massaging balls on your feet and neck can alleviate tension, offering relief from discomfort and promoting relaxation.

<u>While on Holiday</u>

Even during the most leisurely vacation, it's possible to feel overwhelmed and stressed. When planning your trip, incorporate activities specifically designed to enhance self-care.

1. Meditate: Keep a meditation app on your phone to maintain your practice wherever you are.

2. Take walks: Similar to your routine at home, engaging in moderate physical activity will boost blood circulation and elevate endorphin levels.

3. Embrace nature: Regardless of your destination, plan activities that involve being in natural surroundings, as the positive effects of nature have been scientifically proven (refer to Part 6 for more details).

4. Bring your journal: If journaling is part of your self-care routine, ensure you pack it along.

5. Plan a spa visit: Spas are available worldwide, so consider visiting one, even if it's within your hotel.

6. Allow indulgence: Even when traveling on a budget, plan to indulge in one thing, whether it's a luxurious dinner or covering the cost of a checked bag. Continuously stressing about finances throughout the trip will only contribute to anxiety.

Creating a Self-Care Travel Kit

Prepare a self-care-oriented travel kit to ease stress during your journeys and simplify packing. Utilize a compact dopp kit, ensuring it's always stocked with essential self-care items for quick and effortless access. Include the following:
  - Your preferred sheet mask
  - Lavender essential oil in a roller ball

- Hydrating face mist
- High-quality, pleasantly scented hand cream
- Natural sleep aids like melatonin supplements
- Healing ointment for chapped skin and lips
- Cleansing face wipes
- Travel-sized container of your favorite cologne
- CBD tincture or gummies

Mental Health

In contemporary society, prevalent challenges include stress and anxiety, which, if unaddressed, can significantly impact both physical health and mental well-being. Research suggests that reducing stress not only contributes to increased happiness and more fulfilling relationships but also leads to a fuller life. Conversely, neglecting self-care activities may result in severe illnesses, encompassing both physical and mental aspects. Psychologists often use a person's ability to perform self-care tasks, like bathing and oral hygiene, as an indicator for conditions such as anxiety disorders and clinical depression.

Concerning Masculinity and Mental Health, some argue that we are amidst a male mental health crisis, concurrently experiencing a crisis of masculinity. Mental Health America reports that approximately six million men grapple with depression each year. Notably, men are less inclined to seek mental healthcare compared to women, influenced by societal expectations discouraging open discussion of emotions. The notion of the "strong, silent type" as an ideal for men can be detrimental to mental health. Unfortunately, displaying emotions, especially crying, is still often perceived as a feminine trait.

Consequently, a substantial number of mental health issues in men remain undiagnosed annually. Acknowledging the importance of mental health and taking steps to address it is not a sign of weakness; on the contrary, it reflects resilience and strength, showcasing a proactive approach to enhancing one's mental well-being.

Supporting Mental Well-Being through Self-Care

Many mental health challenges in men are often tied to stress, frequently originating from their work environments. A notable number of men express that job-related stress significantly impacts their mental state, persisting even outside working hours. Moreover, anxiety related to employment can detrimentally affect their ability to derive enjoyment from life beyond the workplace. Establishing a positive self-care regimen proves to be a valuable strategy for navigating such stressors, providing a constructive channel for managing aggression and anxiety.

Furthermore, akin to how a positive self-care routine facilitates a connection with one's body, it also fosters an emotional connection. Individuals grappling with depression or those who have experienced abuse may encounter difficulties in tending to their physical well-being. Engaging in self-care aids in reconnecting with one's body and contributes to fostering a positive self-image. Research indicates that individuals proficient in self-care not only exhibit improved stress management but also demonstrate enhanced effectiveness in caring for others.

Tips for Mental Well-Being

To prioritize and enhance your mental health, consider these practical tips and make subtle adjustments to your routine. If you suspect mental health concerns, seeking professional help is advisable.

1. Avoid Isolation:
   - While occasional alone time is beneficial, excessive isolation can negatively impact mental health.
   - Cultivate strong interpersonal relationships for increased happiness.
   - Combat isolation by actively engaging with friends or accepting social invitations.

2. Journaling:
   - Overcome the reluctance to discuss emotions by maintaining a personal journal.
   - Expressing thoughts and feelings in writing promotes constructive emotional processing.
   - Facilitates heightened emotional understanding.

3. Dedicate Daily Time to Yourself:
   - Prioritize self-care daily, even amid other stressors.
   - Engage in activities that bring joy, be it reading, exercising, or pursuing hobbies.
   - The specific activity matters less than its positive impact on your happiness.

4. Practice Gratitude:
   - Adopt gratitude practices for enhanced positive thinking.
   - Maintain a gratitude journal or express affirmations to recognize positive aspects of life.
   - Positively influences outlook and stress management.

5. Limit Smartphone Use:
   - Excessive smartphone reliance fosters isolation and elevates anxiety.
   - Take regular breaks from your phone, disconnecting for short periods.
   - Encourage family members to do the same, promoting face-to-face interactions.

6. Incorporate Exercise:
   - Recognize exercise as a form of self-care for mental health.
   - Moderate physical activity, like a short walk, elevates endorphins, promoting happiness and stress reduction.

7. Practice Forgiveness:
   - Release accumulated daily frustrations to alleviate anxiety.
   - Adopt forgiveness, whether for others or yourself.
   - Cultivate resilience by letting go of minor annoyances and self-blame.

8. Explore Mental Health Apps:
   - Utilize apps dedicated to mental health for cognitive puzzles or therapy resources.
   - Enhance thinking and problem-solving skills through accessible and portable apps.

9. Seek Community:

- Join real-life or online communities to boost happiness and self-esteem.

- Participate in forums, groups, or local events aligned with your interests.

- Establish connections, even with one person, for significant positive impact.

Regarding Therapy

In the past, there was a misconception that seeking therapy implied a personal issue or being labeled as "crazy." It's crucial to discard such outdated views on therapy. Essentially, therapy offers a secure environment where you can openly discuss matters with an unbiased professional, allowing you to express concerns you might not feel comfortable sharing otherwise. Therapy also provides valuable perspectives on life issues that may be challenging to navigate. While therapy is essential for specific concerns like addiction or depression, you don't require a particular reason to start. If hesitant, you can keep it private, and with the convenience of modern therapy apps, you might not even need to leave your home. Hence, there's no valid reason to avoid seeking therapy.

Part 2 : Physical Wellness

In discussions about self-care, there's often a strong focus on external practices that impact the outward appearance of the body. This emphasis on external care, such as indulging in baths or maintaining a skincare routine, isn't without merit. How you tend to the external aspects of your body significantly influences your overall well-being, including your happiness. Activities like baths promote relaxation, and skincare can contribute to a heightened sense of joy.

However, it's crucial to recognize that self-care is a comprehensive journey that extends beyond external appearances. Consider this analogy: meticulously cleaning and beautifying your car's exterior might give it a shiny and new look, but if you neglect the internal maintenance, such as changing the oil, the car won't function optimally. Similarly, your body requires attention to both its external and internal aspects. While the effects of internal care may not be immediately visible, as with having a good hair day, the focus is on how it makes you feel and contributes to your long-term health.

Sleep, an evident component of self-care appreciated by many, is just one facet of a holistic self-care experience. Incorporating supplements can positively influence mood, and aspects like your sex life contribute to overall wellness. Modern options, such as utilizing cannabis for its therapeutic properties rather than solely for recreational purposes, showcase the expanding landscape of self-care possibilities.

To truly elevate your self-care routine, it's essential to examine all facets of your life, extending beyond the contents of your bathroom cabinet. Recognizing the interconnectedness of external and internal well-being ensures a more comprehensive and fulfilling self-care experience.

Supplements

Apart from the childhood multivitamin your mom insisted on, protein powder likely dominates your perception of supplements, a common association for many men. Stepping into a supplement store reveals shelves filled with oversized containers of protein and intense pre-workout blends with names reminiscent of professional wrestlers. Amidst these, smaller jars promise enhancements like improved hair and performance – desires most men share.

Yet, the realm of supplements extends beyond muscle building or sexual wellness. In contemporary times, a new wave of dietary supplements focuses on holistic health, aligning seamlessly with the principles of self-care. Consider this: mushrooms may boost your mood, bacteria can aid in weight loss, and specific proteins might contribute to maintaining youthful skin. It's an intriguing perspective on self-care, showcasing that supplements offer benefits far beyond the traditional notions of muscle enhancement or sexual vitality.

<u>Why Opt for Them?</u>

The pertinent question to consider is, "Why not incorporate

them?" Just as you turn to protein powder for muscle growth, dietary supplements offer a versatile approach to addressing various concerns. The challenge lies in the fact that, unlike protein powder with visible effects, the outcomes of dietary supplements are often intangible. Picture this: consuming protein powder coupled with workouts yields tangible gains swiftly. Conversely, taking a powdered mushroom for stress relief involves effects that are more subjective—an experience rather than a visible transformation. Nevertheless, this doesn't diminish their efficacy.

It's crucial to emphasize that the cornerstone of supplement effectiveness is consistency. In a world driven by quick results, it's essential to acknowledge that several supplements require regular usage for noticeable differences. Sometimes, it's about how you feel rather than observable changes in the mirror. Regularly assess your body to discern any potential shifts and adhere to the recommended dosage; assuming more will yield faster results is a misconception. As with anything health-related, consulting your doctor is prudent if you encounter questions or perceive adverse effects. Not all supplements suit everyone, and discontinuing a supplement that doesn't align with your well-being is a reasonable choice.

<u>Some supplements</u>

Navigating the extensive world of self-care supplements can be overwhelming. When perusing aisles or online platforms, consider exploring these diverse categories to steer you in the right direction.

1. Gut Health Boosters

- Probiotics: These supplements nurture the thousands of bacteria within your body, particularly in the gastrointestinal tract. Supporting "gut flora," they aid digestion, control bloating, and alleviate constipation.

- Prebiotics: Complementary to probiotics, prebiotic supplements act as nourishment for existing gut bacteria, ensuring their vitality and prolonged efficacy. Combining both in a supplement can be a holistic approach to gut health.

2. Adaptogens - Wellness Celebrities

- These supplements, featuring herbs or mushrooms like ashwagandha, reishi, or lion's mane, stand out in the wellness realm for their adaptability to the body's needs. Renowned for reducing inflammation and regulating mood, adaptogens are gaining attention for their stress-reducing properties.

3. Collagen - Beyond Skin Deep

- While known for maintaining skin elasticity, collagen powders transcend cosmetic benefits. Widely used in sports medicine, they aid joint health, enhance recovery from injuries, and contribute to youthful-looking skin across the body.

4. Omega-3 - Cellular Building Blocks

- Omega-3s, commonly associated with fish oil, serve as essential building blocks for various cell types in the body. Though not trend-driven, they play a crucial role in overall health, potentially impacting heart health and mental well-being.

5. Ginkgo Biloba - Brain Booster

- An ancient tree in Chinese herbal medicine, Ginkgo Biloba

has gained popularity in wellness circles. Its antioxidant and anti-inflammatory properties, akin to adaptogens, contribute to brain health, potentially enhancing alertness and memory.

6. Biotin - Hair Strength

- Essential for hair production, biotin, and its counterpart keratin, are now recognized for their potential to promote hair growth when taken orally. Particularly beneficial for men concerned with hair loss, consistent supplementation for at least three months may yield visible effects.

7. Melatonin - Sleep Support

- Not all supplements are morning rituals; melatonin, a natural sleep aid, can enhance sleep quality without resorting to chemical alternatives. While some users report vivid dreams, the side effects are generally milder compared to pharmaceutical sleep aids.

Exercise

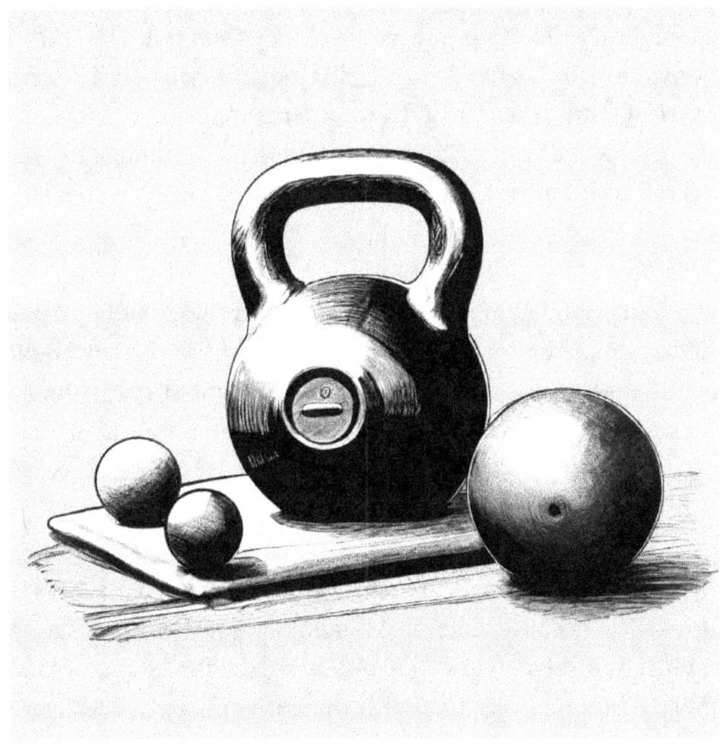

In practical terms, everyone acknowledges the positive impact of exercise on well-being. However, the prevalent perception often revolves around working out solely for aesthetic reasons, as evidenced by the popularity of "fitstagrammers." Undeniably, achieving a healthy body requires effort, but the emphasis has typically been on appearance.

Shifting this perspective, integrating exercise into a self-care routine becomes remarkably accessible, particularly for those already engaged in it. The key lies in a mindset transformation. Rather than viewing exercise through the lens of appearance, consider its effects on how you feel. Beyond crafting a "beach body," research attests to myriad benefits associated with exercise. It's crucial to reframe exercise not as a task to be checked off but as a gratifying activity that contributes to your overall well-being.

This shift might entail disconnecting from Instagram, re-assessing your gym environment, or exploring new classes that resonate better with you. True health isn't solely about achieving specific fitness milestones; it's about cultivating a lifestyle that prioritizes self-care and personal well-being.

<u>Why Incorporating Exercise Matters</u>

If you're questioning the inclusion of exercise in a self-care book, it's because, like any beneficial practice, it offers a multitude of advantages. Notably, these benefits extend beyond mere aesthetics, aligning with the core concept of self-care — how well you're tending to your body's overall health. While regular exercise undoubtedly contributes to an improved appearance, even modest physical activity, such as 20 minutes a day, can significantly enhance various aspects of your life. Here's why:

1. Controls Weight:
   - Moderate exercise plays a fundamental role in weight management. Beyond caloric balance, regular physical activity improves overall body function and reduces fat storage.

2. Helps Prevent Heart Disease:
   - An essential consideration for everyone, moderate exercise proves effective in preventing heart disease. Cardiovascular activities elevate heart rate, strengthening the heart and lowering blood pressure, crucial factors in reducing the risk of heart-related issues.

3. Boosts Energy:
   - Exercise triggers the release of endorphins, hormones in the brain responsible for post-workout energy boosts. It enhances heart function, allowing more efficient oxygen circulation throughout the body, offering a natural remedy for sluggishness.

4. Raises Your Mood:
   - Endorphins not only boost energy but also contribute to an improved mood. These brain chemicals alleviate pain, manage stress, and the more consistently you exercise, the more endorphins are released, fostering a happier state.

5. Promotes Better Sleep:
   - Expending energy during the day through moderate exercise has lasting effects on nighttime sleep quality. Endorphins,

in addition to raising mood and alertness, have been linked to quicker sleep onset and longer periods of rest.

6. Leads to Better Sex:
   - Beyond the confidence boost from feeling physically fit, the sexual benefits of exercise extend to improved blood flow. This increased circulation, vital in preventing heart disease, also enhances overall sexual function, addressing issues like erectile dysfunction.

In essence, exercise is a multifaceted contributor to your well-being, transcending the surface-level focus on appearance and aligning seamlessly with the principles of holistic self-care.

Exercise Tips for Those Averse to the Gym

For individuals not particularly keen on traditional exercise, finding motivation can be challenging. The reality is, there isn't a one-size-fits-all exercise, but any form of physical activity is beneficial for everyone. Prioritizing self-care through exercise doesn't necessitate joining an upscale gym; it can be as straightforward as implementing these small changes:

Dynamic Stretching:
   - Stretching before exercise is crucial for injury prevention, and it can be a form of exercise itself when done right. Active or dynamic stretching involves moving through stretches rather than holding static positions, enhancing flexibility and elevating the heart rate. Try these stretches:
   - Neck Stretch: Tilt your head toward your shoulder without twisting your neck, holding for 15 seconds on each side.

- Lateral Shoulder Stretch: Raise one arm overhead, grasp it with the other hand, and pull the elbow slowly behind the head. Hold for 15 seconds on each side.

- Posterior Shoulder Stretch: Place your right hand on your left shoulder, pull your left arm across the chest toward the right shoulder. Hold for 15 seconds on each side.

- Bridge Stretch: Lift your arms above your head, interlace your fingers if possible, and straighten your elbows. Reach as high as possible, holding for 15 seconds.

Walking:

- With the popularity of wearable fitness devices, walking has gained a new appeal. These devices track steps, encouraging you to make small changes like parking farther away or opting to walk instead of taking the bus.

Take the Stairs:

- Whenever you encounter an elevator, opt for the stairs, especially if it's just a few flights. Climbing stairs provides aerobic exercise, elevating your heart rate and contributing to leg and butt muscle development.

Body Weight Moves:

- Exercise doesn't require fancy machines; body weight movements like push-ups, lunges, and squats are effective in raising your heart rate and building muscle. The convenience lies in their adaptability to various settings.

Ride a Bike:

- Embrace the biking trend in cities as an efficient way to incorporate exercise. Instead of driving or using public transportation, cycling offers aerobic benefits and quicker transportation.

Get an App:

- Modern fitness apps hold you accountable for exercise, providing at-home routines, often focused on body-weight exercises. Set reminders to ensure consistency, especially if scheduling workouts is challenging.

Yoga:

- Yoga, akin to active stretching, improves flexibility while increasing the heart rate. Its minimal impact nature makes it suitable for individuals with joint issues, and studies suggest potential benefits for insomnia.

Detoxification

At its core, detoxification or cleansing aims to eliminate toxins from your body. These toxins aren't limited to substances like drugs or alcohol, although we use similar terminology. They can originate from various sources such as environmental pollution, chemicals, preservatives, pesticides in your food, and more. The concept revolves around the idea that your body can accumulate various toxins, impacting its optimal functionality. Through detoxing, you essentially purify your system, flushing out accumulated toxins. Typically, this involves fasting or adhering to a strict diet for a defined period, allowing your body to eliminate anything harmful.

Most detox programs focus on the liver, kidneys, and gut, acting as your body's filtration system, which can become congested, much like a shower drain. A detox cleanse aids in expelling undesirable substances from these areas, facilitating more effective filtration. Consider it as a Drano for your body, ensuring a thorough purification process.

<u>Why Undertake It?</u>

Advocates of cleansing argue that regular detoxes enable their bodies to operate at an elevated level. At times, toxins can accumulate in people's bodies gradually, and they may not even recognize that they're experiencing discomfort. Perhaps you're dealing with unexplained chronic headaches, enduring a prolonged period of sluggishness, facing challenges in your regular workouts, feeling unusually bloated, or experiencing worsened allergies. The notion behind a detox cleanse is that it could potentially help you feel better by essentially resetting your body. However, your motivation for undertaking a cleanse doesn't need to be extensively planned. Whether you indulged a bit too much on vacation, overindulged at a friend's bachelor party, or simply want to shake off the aftermath of a night out – that's a valid reason too.

Key Considerations Before Starting

Before embarking on any cleanse, it is essential to consult your doctor. They can assess whether you have any underlying health issues that need consideration during the cleansing process. Keep in mind that not everyone embraces the concept of cleanses, so approach their advice with an open mind. If you decide to proceed with the cleanse, regardless of its type, anticipate potential side effects. It's normal to experience irritability, moodiness, lethargy, or even flu-like symptoms in the initial days. These reactions are part of your body undergoing withdrawal from substances it might be accustomed to, such as sugar and carbs. The more indulgent your lifestyle before the cleanse, the more challenging it might be.

Crucially, cleanses yield results only if consistently adhered to, so choose a plan that aligns with your commitment level.

If you're new to cleansing, consider starting with a shorter duration, like a couple of days, before attempting an extended regimen like a three-week juice cleanse. This approach allows you to gauge your comfort and satisfaction with the process.

Varieties of Detox Cleanses

All detox cleanses share a common objective: removing undesirable elements from your diet. The method you choose to achieve this goal is flexible.

Juice Cleanse:
   - This popular detox involves abstaining from solid food and exclusively consuming fresh juices. Typically lasting from a few days to a few weeks, you'll drink five or six juices daily. While providing nourishment, some may find it challenging due to the absence of chewing sensations (certain cleanses permit low-calorie foods like celery).

Fasting:
   - The original detox method where you refrain from consuming any food for a specified duration. Contemporary approaches include intermittent fasting, limiting eating to a set daily window, or specific food consumption only at night. The idea is to reset your body to rely on stored nutrients instead of constant intake.

Elimination Diet:
   - These diets involve a highly restricted intake, often limited to lean proteins and specific vegetables. Initially designed to identify food allergies, they are now utilized in detoxing,

particularly for those concerned about reactions to substances like gluten or sugar.

Colon Cleanse:
  - Targeting the colon and GI tract, this cleanse addresses issues like constipation and bloating. It comes in various forms, from high-fiber shakes to drinking salt water. Supervision by a medical professional is advisable to prevent potential GI tract damage.

Liver Cleanse:
  - Focused on the liver, this cleanse is appealing to those with alcohol-heavy lifestyles. It often incorporates a restricted or juice diet along with additional supplements. However, scientific evidence regarding its effectiveness is inconclusive.

Bone Broth Cleanse:
  - Similar to fasting or juice cleanses, this program restricts your diet to exclusively drinking bone broth, popularized by the Paleo movement. Usually lasting a few days, it aims to reset your body while providing essential nutrients and protein.

BOWEL MOVEMENTS

In straightforward terms, experiencing challenges with bowel movements can be a concern during a cleanse. This is primarily due to the limited fiber content in juice or broth diets, and in the case of fasting, the absence of food intake results in reduced fiber and less waste to eliminate. Some individuals opt for colonics during their cleanse to assist in clearing any blockages and maintaining regular bowel movements. Alternatively, some navigate the lack of flow and anticipate improved conditions post-cleanse. It's crucial not to exert force; rather, allow natural bowel movements to occur. A helpful tip: after completing the cleanse, initiate with easily digestible, fiber-rich foods to ensure smooth digestive processes. Occasionally, during a juice cleanse, increased bowel movements may occur as the body effectively eliminates accumulated waste and toxins. Regardless, the ultimate aim is toxin removal, making it a worthwhile endeavor.

Sleep

How often have you uttered the phrase, "I'll sleep when I'm dead," prioritizing activities like partying or working over a restful night's sleep? Sleep might seem inconsequential, particularly in youth, but it plays a crucial role in bodily functions. During sleep, your body undergoes repair, produces essential hormones for development, and enhances brain function. Contrary to the notion that sleep is for the weak, inadequate sleep can have both physical and mental repercussions, resulting in decreased energy, weakened cognitive abilities, and potential long-term health issues such as heart failure and strokes. Conditions like insomnia and untreated sleep apnea can even pose life-threatening risks.

These effects are likely familiar, experienced after a hectic workweek or a party-filled vacation. Establishing a healthy sleep routine, ensuring sufficient sleep time, is a fundamental aspect of any self-care regimen. In reality, many self-care principles aim to promote relaxation, ultimately facilitating better sleep. Sleeping amidst stress proves challenging, making self-care an effective means of stress relief. The initial step involves shifting the perspective on sleep – transforming it from a mandatory task to a crucial bodily need, and perhaps eventually, a desirable activity.

Deep sleep

Deep sleep is the fourth and deepest stage in the human sleep cycle. During this phase, the body undergoes significant restorative processes. The muscles relax, breathing slows down, and both heart rate and body temperature decrease. This crucial stage is when the body engages in healing activities, including tissue repair, the production and release of essential hormones, and the formation of memories and learning processing by the brain.

Research suggests that approximately 23 percent of nightly sleep, equivalent to around 90 minutes, should be dedicated to deep sleep. However, reaching this stage requires progressing through the preceding three sleep stages, necessitating several hours of quality sleep. Individuals with sleep-related issues like insomnia or sleep apnea may struggle to attain this phase. Without sufficient deep sleep, the body lacks the necessary time for rebuilding, leading to symptoms of sleep deprivation such as mental fog and fatigue.

Enhancing Your Sleep Routine

Whether you're a sound sleeper or struggle with sleep, establishing a positive bedtime routine, known as "sleep hygiene," can have a significant impact. Consider it as important as your daily shower.

1. Dim the Lights: Ensure your bedroom has low and calming lighting. If exposed to excessive natural or city light, consider

blackout curtains. Opt for curtains or blinds that filter light if you prefer waking up to natural light.

2. Lower the Temperature: Maintain a cool room, possibly around 60°F, as deep sleep is associated with a decrease in body temperature.

3. Limit Screen Time: Blue light from screens can disrupt relaxation. Turn off all screens at least an hour before bedtime. Charge your phone in another room and consider removing TVs from the bedroom.

4. Avoid Stimulants: Reduce caffeine intake in the afternoon, allowing your body to process it before bedtime.

5. Start Your Routine Earlier: Develop a bedtime routine an hour before sleeping, involving activities like teeth brushing, face washing, a relaxing bath, meditation, or stretching.

6. Don't Eat Too Late: Consider not eating after 8 p.m., allowing for better digestion and avoiding issues like acid reflux. Choose a time at least 2 hours before bedtime.

7. Invest in Quality Sheets: Opt for sheets that regulate body temperature, like linen, which may keep you cooler. Cotton is a good standard, but use an unscented detergent if you have sensitive skin.

8. Use a Noise Machine: Combat noise pollution, especially in urban environments, by using earplugs or a white noise machine to mask disruptive sounds during the night.

Water

Nighttime cramps, often occurring in the legs and experienced by up to 60 percent of adults, lack a fully understood explanation. Dehydration is considered a potential factor, and maintaining proper hydration during the day may yield improvement. However, guzzling a large glass of water before bedtime may not be the ideal solution, especially if it leads to nocturnal bathroom trips. This creates a dilemma: waking due to leg cramps or waking to urinate, both disrupting the sleep cycle. One alternative is to ensure consistent water intake throughout the day. Another option involves a homeopathic approach—consuming a shot of pickle brine before sleep. The theory suggests that the brine's salt content aids water retention overnight, keeping the limbs hydrated.

Part 3: The Body

When considering body care, the emphasis often falls on internal aspects. While internal health is undoubtedly crucial, the impact of caring for the external aspects of your body is equally significant.

General hygiene transcends mere necessity; it holds substantial implications for long-term health. Yet, its effects extend beyond physical well-being. The actions you take for your body significantly influence mental health and mood. Aromatherapy, for example, operates on the premise that specific scents can modify brain chemistry, promoting relaxation, improving sleep, or providing an energizing effect. Consequently, aromatherapy finds application in various practices such as baths, massages, and personal care products like lotions and oils.

Self-care for the body goes beyond relaxation. Consider tattoos—an intentional act to shape the body according to your desires. This desire lies at the heart of self-care: engaging in activities that contribute to becoming the person you aspire to be. Whether your objectives involve a physical transformation or simply maintaining freshness, proper body care stands out as one of the most beneficial practices.

Baths not showers

You might not have indulged in a bath since childhood, and there's a reason for that. Baths represent a commitment— showers are functional and quick, while baths demand dedicating what may feel like an unnecessary amount of time. Moreover, in a world increasingly fixated on screens, deliberately engaging in an activity that restricts screen use can seem like a form of self-inflicted torment.

These aspects are precisely why baths have become a cornerstone of the self-care movement. They compel you to carve out time from your busy life and engage in a solitary activity, unless, of course, you're using a bath for more intimate purposes. Baths are inherently private, urging you to be alone with your thoughts, devoid of distractions. Additionally, baths are incredibly relaxing, often conjuring images of rose-petal-filled tubs surrounded by an abundance of candles, resembling a serene vigil. While some people go all out with their baths, you don't need an entire book of matches and an Enya album to enjoy the benefits.

And what are these benefits? They extend well beyond cleanliness. Ever heard the advice, "To get really clean, take a bath"? It's true—immersing yourself in water for an extended period is unparalleled for cleanliness. However, when it comes to baths for self-care, the rationale transcends mere hygiene. Baths can bring about tangible changes in your mood, internal bodily functions, and long-term health.

<u>The Wellness Advantages of Baths</u>

Bathing has served as a fundamental element of wellness in various cultures for centuries. The Japanese, in particular, have a term for wellness-oriented bathing: onsen. Their knowledge, backed increasingly by science, underscores that bathing can effectively address diverse health issues.

Elevate Your Mood

Certain studies suggest that immersing your body in water can evoke sensations reminiscent of being in a womb, fostering feelings of comfort and security. These studies also indicate that bathing may alleviate anxiety, reduce depression, and mitigate feelings of pessimism.

Muscle Recovery

Frequent sightings of bathtubs in sports medicine offices have a reason: hot baths enhance circulation, alleviating muscle pain and loosening tight muscles. Conversely, ice-cold baths constrict blood vessels, aiding in reducing swelling and expediting muscle regeneration.

Enhance Sleep Quality

As the body temperature decreases during sleep, melatonin—a natural sleep aid—is produced. Taking a hot bath before bedtime is believed to expedite this process by raising body temperature, facilitating the internal temperature drop conducive to sleep.

Reinforce Your Immune System

Apart from relieving congestion, the steam from a hot bath and the warm water itself may contribute to disease prevention. Studies indicate that certain immune system cells operate more efficiently at higher temperatures induced by a bath.

Promote Heart Health

Regular hot baths have shown effectiveness in reducing blood pressure. The heat promotes increased blood flow and circulation, lowering blood pressure and decreasing the risk of heart attack and stroke.

Caloric Expenditure

Research suggests that the cardiovascular effects of increased blood flow during a hot bath are comparable to exercise. Hot baths elevate heart rate and induce sweating, potentially burning calories equivalent to a brisk walk.

Soothe the Skin

Warm baths, combined with essential oils and soothing ingredients, have demonstrated efficacy in reducing skin inflammation associated with conditions like eczema, psoriasis, and sunburn. They also provide comprehensive hydration, surpassing the effects of creams and lotions, although excessively hot baths can have a drying effect.

Alleviate Arthritis Discomfort

The muscle-relaxing properties of hot baths extend to loosening stiff joints. The addition of Epsom salt, readily absorbed through hot water, can aid in pain management and further assist in lubricating rigid joints.

Crafting the Ideal Bath

Now that you're aware of the advantages of a bath, let's delve into the essentials for creating the perfect one:

1. Water: This is a given. Ensure it's not excessively hot to prevent burns.

2. Salt: Especially Epsom salt, known for its muscle-soothing properties, mineral absorption promotion, and relaxation facilitation.

3. Essential Oils: Apart from having distinct properties when absorbed through the skin, certain essential oils contribute to sleep promotion or healing. Additionally, their scents offer added aromatherapy benefits.

4. Oatmeal: Opt for colloidal oatmeal commonly found in bathing products. This type, ground and suspended in liquid, is particularly effective in soothing skin ailments.

5. Baking Soda: Even the baking soda from your kitchen cabinet can serve as a potent exfoliator, aiding in the removal of calluses and dead skin.

6. Ice Cubes: While ice-cold baths might not be as immediately

relaxing, they can prove beneficial for muscle recovery and post-workout healing.

Activities for Your Bath Time

While you're in the bath, take advantage of your free time by engaging in the following:

1. Read: Grab an actual book, not your iPad, and immerse yourself in a good read.

2. Reflect: Utilize this moment to decompress from your day and engage in thoughtful contemplation.

3. Meditate: The tranquility of the bath provides an ideal setting to clear your mind through meditation.

4. Tend to Your Fingernails: Take the opportunity to clean and care for your fingernails — a task often overlooked.

5. Listen to Music: Enjoy some music, ensuring that the speaker is positioned at a safe distance from the water.

Pedicures and Manicures

Taking care of your hands and feet is more than just about meeting your partner's expectations; it's an essential aspect of self-care. While many women express their preference for well-maintained nails and smooth feet in a man, the primary motivation for manicures and pedicures should be personal well-being. In this judgment-free zone, your individual reasons for considering nail, hand, and foot maintenance are valid. Ultimately, the key to self-care lies in recognizing the importance of caring for these often-overlooked body parts.

Hands, being the most utilized tools, play a crucial role in daily life, while feet silently bear significant burdens. Discomfort or pain in these areas can substantially impact your overall well-being. Whether your hands are frequently exposed or your livelihood depends on them, proper care is essential. Similarly, if you wear sandals or go barefoot, maintaining the health and cleanliness of your feet is crucial.

Manicures and pedicures extend beyond aesthetics; they contribute to the cleanliness and health of your most-used appendages. Beyond the tangible benefits, the experience itself is immensely enjoyable. Professional services offer a level of care that's challenging to replicate at home, providing a relaxing and rejuvenating experience. While professional sessions are affordable and low-risk, you can also incorporate self-manicures and pedicures into your routine for effective self-care. The key is to prioritize this practice for the overall well-being of your hands and feet.

Why Opt for a Manicure?

While maintaining neatly trimmed and clean fingernails enhances your overall appearance, there are substantial health benefits associated with getting a manicure. Regularly tending to your fingernails by trimming and cleaning contributes to their strength, preventing brittleness and avoiding issues like ingrown nails. Moreover, this practice helps fend off the growth of bacteria and fungus, preventing potential long-term problems with your fingers and nails. Consistent moisturizing of cuticles serves to prevent hangnails and promotes healthy nail growth. Professional manicures often include a hand massage, promoting improved blood circulation and inducing relaxation throughout your entire body, thanks to the pressure points in your hands. Some manicures also incorporate exfoliation to eliminate dead skin and prevent the formation of calluses.

What Does a Pedicure Involve?

Pedicures adhere to a similar process as manicures, but they focus on your feet. For men who often overlook foot care more than hand care, pedicures become especially crucial. Feet, being potential breeding grounds for bacteria, are particularly important to address, especially if you frequently walk barefoot on tile floors or wear sandals. Enclosed in shoes for much of the time, feet create a favorable environment for bacteria and fungi to thrive due to darkness and moisture. Neglecting proper foot care may lead to issues such as ingrown toenails, elevating the risk of painful bacterial infections. Conditions like athlete's foot, caused by a fungus, can become itchy and uncomfortable if not promptly treated. Additionally, there's a risk of developing serious skin cancers like melanoma and basal cell carcinoma on the feet. While a pedicure isn't a cure for cancer, it could contribute to early detection. Notably, Bob Marley succumbed to an unchecked melanoma on his foot.

Manicure/Pedicure Procedure Steps

The standard procedure for most manicures and pedicures is consistent, with or without nail polish. Here's what you can typically expect:

1. Clean:
   - The technician begins by cleaning the surface of your nails to eliminate dirt, and if necessary, cleans underneath them.

2. Cut:
   - Using a nail clipper, your nails are cut to the desired length and shaped, often rounded.

3. File:
   - Following the nail cutting, a nail file is used to smooth the ends, ensuring they are even and not rough.

4. Soak:

- You might be asked to dip your fingertips in a liquid bowl to moisturize the nails and cuticles. Cuticle oil may be applied for additional hydration.

5. Push:

- Optionally, the technician may use a tool to gently push the cuticle skin away from the nail surface, facilitating easier trimming, particularly beneficial if you struggle with hangnails.

6. Moisturize:

- Depending on your needs, the technician might apply a scrub to exfoliate your hands, followed by the application of moisturizing cream. This step often includes a relaxing hand massage.

7. Buff:

- If you prefer a polish-free look, you can choose to have your nails buffed for a shiny and healthy appearance. Alternatively, you can opt for nail polish, either clear or colored, based on your preference.

DIY Pedicure at Home

If the idea of a public pedicure isn't appealing, you can pamper your feet at home with these steps:

1. Immerse your feet in a warm water and Epsom salt bath for approximately 10 minutes. This soak aids in softening your skin and calluses, making exfoliation easier.

2. While still soaking, utilize a foot scrub to exfoliate dead skin and eliminate calluses. Use a pumice stone to smooth away any remaining calluses.

3. Trim your toenails using a straight-edge clipper, ensuring not to cut them excessively short to avoid pain and the risk of fungal issues.

4. File the edges of your nails with a nail file or emery board to maintain a smooth finish.

5. Apply a moisturizing foot cream generously over your feet, including between your toes, and ensure thorough rubbing for complete absorption.

Skin care

Prioritizing proper skin care is a crucial aspect of your self-care routine, not only for maintaining a great appearance but also to safeguard your skin from potential issues in the future. This principle extends to the care of the skin on your body, recognizing subtle differences from facial skin, such as thickness, oil production, and hair follicles. Despite these distinctions, fundamental skincare practices remain applicable.

Contrary to women, most men are not educated about caring for their bodies, leaving their skin susceptible to aging and other concerns related to inflammation and dehydration. Often, men tend to neglect the skin below their necks, largely due to negative perceptions of lotions. Many view lotions as akin to sunscreen—goopy, messy, and uncomfortable, resulting in an aversion to regular use. This perspective, in part, stems from associating lotions with fixing issues like chapped hands instead of preventing them.

The misconception that a soft hand isn't masculine contributes to men viewing body moisturizing as a reactionary measure rather than a preventive one. However, self-care doesn't compromise masculinity; rather, it reflects confidence and strength in understanding and meeting one's body's health needs.

Effectively caring for your body involves simple steps like changing your body wash and finding a lotion with a tolerable scent. Consistency is paramount, as many men tend to use products like lotion only when they feel a specific need, delaying the effectiveness. Once you identify a lotion or body oil you find agreeable, incorporating it into your routine consistently becomes one of the simplest yet impactful self-care practices.

Importance of skin care

Extending your skincare routine beyond your face to encompass your torso, arms, hands, and even lower regions is essential for similar reasons you care for your facial skin. Practices like exfoliation and hydration not only enhance the immediate appearance of your skin, especially if adorned with tattoos (discussed later), but also ensure optimal functionality of the skin cells on your body. To achieve this, the skin requires turnover through exfoliation, hydration via moisturizing, and maintenance of cleanliness through washing.

Men are susceptible to inflammatory skin issues on their bodies, such as eczema and psoriasis, characterized by chronic dryness, itching, flaking, and irritation. Neglecting proper skincare exacerbates these concerns, while incorporating measures like using lotions and appropriate cleansers can mitigate their impact. For individuals dealing with eczema and psoriasis, seeking guidance from a doctor is advisable for comprehensive management, recognizing that gentle, unscented lotion serves as just the initial step. Even for men without these specific issues but who occasionally face dry skin due to activities like outdoor sports, tending to the skin on the body plays a pivotal role in addressing such conditions.

What you should do

Here's a simplified skincare routine for your body that doesn't involve numerous steps:

Cleanse:

Opt for a gentle cleanser designed for sensitive skin, avoiding products that leave your skin overly stripped. Charcoal-infused options can help absorb dirt effectively, but be cautious with ingredients like tea tree and peppermint oil, especially if you have sensitive skin.

Exfoliate:

Consider using a loofah sponge or a body scrub with salicylic acid occasionally to eliminate dead skin cells, particularly beneficial for those prone to body acne (folliculitis).

Lotion:

After showering, apply a lightweight, fragrance-free moisturizing lotion to lock in moisture and keep your skin hydrated. This is especially useful for individuals with dry skin or chronic issues like eczema.

Oil:

If lotions aren't preferred, explore body oils containing natural ingredients and essential oils. These oils provide hydration and fast absorption, best used right after a shower.

Unlike lotions, oils soften skin by retaining moisture but don't draw moisture from the air into your skin.

WHAT IS CHAFING?

Every man has encountered chafing – when unprotected skin, such as underarms, between buttocks, or inner thighs, rubs together, resulting in dry and irritated skin. This is particularly common during physical activity when skin friction is more frequent and prolonged. Chafing ranges from discomfort to potentially causing lesions that may become infected. The key to prevention is regularly applying a lotion with zinc oxide, forming a protective barrier on the skin. Specialized chafing products, like sticks and lotions, utilize powders and other ingredients to enhance "slip," preventing skin friction.

Tan

Having a sun-kissed complexion serves as a symbol of status, suggesting that one has enjoyed outdoor activities instead of being confined to a desk. Additionally, a tan is often associated with good health, contrasting with the subconscious link between paleness and illness. This is particularly relevant for men, as our culture still values the ruggedness associated with an active lifestyle. Despite the awareness of the risks, such as sun damage, premature aging, and skin cancer due to UV rays, the desire for a tan persists. The allure of a tan lies in its ability to conceal imperfections, create a smoother skin appearance, and even act as a real-life Photoshop to mask blemishes. Striking a balance between the cultural preference for tan skin and the awareness of its harmful effects presents a challenging dilemma.

How to Get it

To comprehend the potential risks of tanning, it's essential to grasp the process of how one develops a tan. The sun's UV rays penetrate the outer skin layer, stimulating the production of melanin—the compound responsible for dark pigment and preventing skin from burning. This melanin production is what accounts for varying skin tones. As melanin accumulates, the skin gradually darkens. However, there's a limit to the amount of melanin the body can generate, and once that threshold is reached, sunburn occurs, irrespective of the amount of sunscreen applied.

Why is it bad

The melanin production itself is not problematic, but exceeding the body's natural limits becomes a concern. Once your innate defenses are depleted, UV rays begin damaging the DNA of your cells. The body responds by increasing blood flow to aid in cell repair, leading to painful sunburn in the short term and potentially mutated cells causing skin cancer in the long term. UV rays also generate free radicals, small molecules that steal electrons from others, causing damage linked to skin cancer and premature aging. While UV-induced sun damage is inevitable, deliberately harming the skin for a tan treads a perilous path.

How to Safely Achieve a Tan

Despite the potential harm from UV rays, the desire for a tan persists. Fortunately, there are safer and quicker methods than basking on a beach.

1. Wear Sunscreen:

Protect yourself from the sun's damaging rays by wearing sunscreen daily, especially on your face. This essential practice is crucial when spending extended periods outdoors. While you'll still get a tan, it might take longer. Opt for sunscreen with SPF 30 or higher.

2. Sunless Tanning:

Sunless tanning products containing dihydroxyacetone (DHA) react with dead skin cells, providing a temporary darkening effect. Although it doesn't replicate the natural melanin-producing process and doesn't last as long, it offers a tan appearance without the risk of future skin cancer. Sunless tanning products come in various forms like sprays, mousses, creams, and drops, with consistent use building the desired color.

3. Bronzer:

Bronzers offer a quick, temporary tan solution, especially for the face. Available in powder, gel, and cream forms, they provide an instant tan effect. Gels, particularly suitable for most men, can be applied alone or mixed with a moisturizer. Begin with a small amount, adding more for additional color. Be cautious with the application on your neck, especially if wearing light-colored clothing. Remember to wash your face at the end of the day to prevent buildup in pores and stains on pillowcases.

<u>Using Sunless Tanning Products Effectively</u>

To achieve a natural-looking tan with sunless tanning products, it's crucial to follow the proper application steps:

1. Exfoliate First:

Before applying sunless tanner, exfoliate the targeted areas thoroughly to remove dead skin cells, ensuring a more uniform result.

2. Ensure You're Completely Dry:

Apply sunless tanner to dry skin for an even appearance, as water can dilute the product and lead to spotting or streaks.

3. Massage In the Product:

Utilize circular motions to massage the product into the desired tan areas, ensuring thorough absorption into the skin.

4. Be Careful on Your Joints:

Exercise caution on drier areas like elbows and knees, as they tend to absorb more self-tanner. Apply with a lighter touch in these regions.

5. Wash Your Hands:

After application, wash your hands thoroughly to prevent them from appearing dirty or orange due to leftover product.

6. Follow the Directions:

Different products have varying application times. Adhere to the recommended time, which can range from a few minutes to overnight.

7. Dry Before Dressing:

Allow your body to dry completely before dressing to minimize the risk of uneven results.

8. Moisturize Daily:

Once the tan has dried, maintain skin hydration with daily use of lotion or cream. Dehydration is detrimental to any tan, whether natural or sunless.

9. Get Professional Help:

If the process seems daunting, consider a professional spray tan. Utilize online review sites and examine before-and-after pictures to identify a provider with exemplary results.

AVOID TANNING BEDS

In the past, there was a misconception that indoor tanning was safer than sun exposure. However, scientific understanding now contradicts this belief. Tanning beds employ highly concentrated UV rays to accelerate skin tanning, surpassing the natural sunlight pace. Due to infrequent sunscreen use among tanning bed users, skin damage can occur more rapidly compared to sunbathing. The American Academy of Dermatology emphasizes that even a single session of indoor tanning significantly elevates the risk of all skin cancers, particularly if initiated before the age of thirty-five. According to the Centers for Disease Control and Prevention, preventing individuals under eighteen from using tanning beds could avert 61,839 melanomas and 6,735 melanoma-related deaths across the lifetime of 61.2 million children. The compelling evidence has led the FDA to mandate warning labels on all indoor tanning devices.

Spa Day

For some reason, many men don't consider spas as practical tools for their own self-care. Culturally, spas are often viewed as luxurious retreats reserved for occasional pampering, and there's a perception that they are predominantly feminine—private havens where women relax in towels and undergo treatments like mud baths. In the minds of numerous men, spas can seem intimidating, peculiar, and uncomfortable.

Contrary to these notions, spas are incredibly appealing. They are not only enjoyable and relaxing but also serve as valuable tools for self-care. Everyone should experience a spa at least once in their life willingly and openly, and it's almost certain that the experience will leave you eager to return.

Spas can be likened to theme parks for self-care, offering a diverse range of treatments such as facials, massages, steam rooms, and even unique features like floatation chambers and rooms constructed from Himalayan salt. Similar to theme parks, the spa experience can either be the time of your life or potentially overwhelming. The key lies in understanding what you seek from it. Done right, a spa visit will leave you revitalized, enthusiastic, and eager for a return trip.

<u>Why Bother?</u>

Drawing on the analogy, your bathroom is akin to a high school carnival, but a spa is the equivalent of Disney World. The level of relaxation achieved in a spa environment is unparalleled. While some individuals visit spas without engaging in specific activities, most go for distinct experiences like massages or facials—services that cannot be replicated at home. At their essence, spas provide services that elevate your self-care routine to a whole new level.

<u>How to Select a Spa</u>

The most straightforward method for choosing a spa is not to choose at all. If you're staying at a hotel with a spa, allocate some time to explore it. Hotel spas are typically uncomplicated, less crowded, and often free for guests. Take advantage of amenities like the steam room or sauna to gauge your liking for the experience.

For those in urban or suburban areas, explore local day spas. Visit their websites to review the services and amenities they offer, and check whether appointments are necessary. Examine the price list, ensuring it aligns with your budget, as some spas can be pricey. Delve into online reviews for insights into others' experiences, focusing on cleanliness, staff friendliness and professionalism, and the overall atmosphere. Spa employees should create a welcoming environment, so feel free to ask questions when booking your appointment, especially if it's your first time. They can provide a tour and address any concerns. Always verify that therapists and providers are licensed.

What to Experience During Your Visit

The versatility of most spas allows you to tailor your experience to your preferences. A typical day spa provides a menu of options, ranging from facials and massages to body treatments and more. Some spas offer additional amenities like soaking pools, saunas, and steam rooms, accessible even without a treatment (common in hotel spas). Certain establishments allow you to purchase time to use their facilities independently.

Spas are often co-ed, but there are male-only options if that's more comfortable. Upon arrival, you'll be directed to a locker room for a robe and sandals (check the spa's dress code in advance). Single-sex saunas, steam rooms, and showers are typically located in the locker room. Outside, a waiting area awaits you, where you'll await your treatment. Depending on your chosen service, your therapist will guide you to the appropriate room.

Communal areas like soaking pools, hot tubs, saunas, and steam rooms are generally available for use, even without a treatment. In these areas, you'll find people lounging, soaking in baths, and indulging in relaxation.

Understanding the Spa Service Menu

While spa treatments can vary across locations, most spas offer variations of these fundamental services. The spa's menu typically provides detailed descriptions specific to that establishment.

1. Massage:

Massages, encompassing a range like deep tissue, hot stone, Thai, and shiatsu, are iconic spa treatments. If you're new to massages, consider starting with a classic Swedish massage. Spas usually allow you to choose between a male or female therapist.

2. Facial:

Facials, once exclusive to spas, remain integral to many spa offerings. Refer to Part 4 for more details on the importance of facials.

3. Body Wrap:

Body treatments, including wraps, act like facials for your entire body. Most wraps involve applying moisturizing creams or lotions before wrapping you in a sheet or blanket, facilitating deeper cream absorption and leaving your skin soft.

4. Body Scrub:

Similar to wraps, scrubs are body treatments where an exfoliant is applied to remove dead skin cells, followed by moisturizer.

5. Manicure/Pedicure:

Spa manicures or pedicures typically focus more on moisturizing and relaxation than those at local nail salons, but the steps are generally similar.

6. Amenities:

General spa amenities like steam rooms, saunas, soaking pools, Jacuzzi-style baths, and occasionally special showers are usually available without specific booking, considered as extra perks.

The Face

In the realm of self-care and personal grooming, there is significant overlap in the Venn diagram. Men often view grooming as a functional necessity—ensuring cleanliness, presenting acceptable hair appearance for public outings, and shaving to avoid resembling Grizzly Adams (unless intentionally embracing that look). However, grooming serves not only utilitarian purposes but is also a means of enhancing personal well-being.

Consider the soap you choose; it's not solely about cleaning efficacy. Soap selection involves factors like fragrance, the post-use feel on your skin, and even its aesthetic appeal in your shower. While self-care may conjure images of spa visits and time-consuming activities, initiating a self-care routine can begin with small, simple actions that bring joy. Caring for your face, a prominent aspect of personal presentation, can be one of these uplifting practices.

A well-groomed face serves as your calling card, instilling confidence and perhaps even a sense of swagger. Research indicates that feeling good about one's appearance has a tangible positive impact on mood and confidence. Anyone who has experienced the boost of confidence from a good hair day can attest to the truth of this phenomenon.

ESTABLISHING A SKINCARE ROUTINE

Many men neglect proper skincare, citing reasons such as lack of time, uncertainty about skincare practices, or perceived notions of it being too feminine. It's time to discard these excuses; taking care of your skin is not only permissible but crucial. The skin, your body's largest organ, deserves attention, with facial skin being particularly important due to its frequent exposure to external elements.

A skincare routine is an uncomplicated yet effective form of self-care, contributing not only to an improved appearance but also to an enhanced sense of well-being. Similar to a morning cup of coffee perking you up, a skincare routine can invigorate you in the morning, while a nighttime routine aids relaxation.

The cornerstone of any skincare routine is realism. Avoid overwhelming yourself with an extensive regimen initially; simplicity is key. Immediate improvements will be noticeable, but consistency is the linchpin to an effective skincare routine.

The Basics:
If, like many men, you primarily wash your face with water and haven't used a moisturizer, here are the initial steps to build a skincare routine.

1. Use a Facial Cleanser:
Opt for a facial cleanser designed to clean effectively without

disturbing your face's delicate pH balance. A tight, dry feeling after washing indicates harsh soap; choose a gentle facial cleanser for both morning and night use.

- Recommended Products: Choose a product labeled "gentle" or, if specific skin issues exist, opt for formulas targeting those concerns, such as sensitive skin or acne-fighting formulas.

2. Follow with an Eye Cream:
   Signs of aging often manifest around the eyes (dark circles, bags, and droopy lids). Combat these issues with an eye cream, loaded with ingredients addressing various concerns. Even if wrinkles aren't a current concern, starting early is beneficial.

- Recommended Products: Seek eye creams containing caffeine for skin energization and peptides for skin-building proteins. Gel formulas are an alternative for those averse to creams.

3. Finish with a Moisturizer:
   Dehydrated skin appears dull, but well-moisturized skin looks healthier and ages more gracefully. Like keeping your gas tank full, moisturize morning and night after applying eye cream.

- Recommended Products: Opt for lightweight gels or lotions to avoid a heavy feeling. If you have oily skin, choose an oil-free formula labeled "matte." Ideally, select a moisturizer with SPF for added sun protection.

Elevated Techniques

Having mastered the fundamentals of your skincare routine, you can now enhance your regimen with a few advanced steps.

Level Up with Serum:

Serums function as power-ups in Super Mario Bros, providing specific advantages. These concentrated formulations, featuring ingredients like brightening vitamin C or moisture-retaining hyaluronic acid, should be applied after cleansing in both your morning and nighttime routines.

- Recommended Products: Start with a serum targeting multiple aspects. Opt for ingredients like hyaluronic acid, vitamin B, and peptides, which contribute to cellular-level skin improvement and play a crucial role in skin regeneration.

Exfoliate Smarter:

Unbeknownst to many, you're likely exfoliating while shaving. The razor's blade sloughs away dead skin cells, making exfoliation vital to prevent the accumulation of dead cells on your skin surface and potential pore blockages. Even if you shave, regularly exfoliate your entire face.

- Recommended Products: While facial scrubs are acceptable, they can be harsh. Instead, choose a chemical exfoliant with alpha hydroxy acids (e.g., glycolic acid) for a gentler removal of dead cells.

Night Cream Is the Right Cream:

For optimal skin health, incorporating a night cream is advisable. During the day, your skin faces various aggressors such as sunlight, pollution, and dirt. At night, when cells are not actively combating these elements, they regenerate. Night creams support this regeneration process.

- Recommended Products: Select a night cream with active ingredients like hydrating hyaluronic acid, anti-aging retinol, or tone-enhancing ceramides. If you prefer a lighter feel, consider using an oil instead of a heavy cream.

Your Shopping Guide

Where to Shop:
   Quality skincare is readily available; you just need to know where to explore. Start at your local big box or drugstore for accessible options. While department stores may seem daunting, their salespeople can provide assistance. Consider the internet, where numerous large online retailers feature dedicated men's grooming sections.

Budget Considerations:
   If you're new to skincare, there's no need to spend extravagantly. Drugstore products can be as effective as luxury ones. Save on items like facial cleansers, while considering a splurge on serums and eye creams.

Quality Assessment:
   When shopping online, leverage user reviews for insights into product effectiveness. Keep in mind that skin types vary, so seek advice from salespeople if shopping in person.

Simplified Approach:
   For those unsure where to start, look for boxed sets. Some

brands offer conveniently bundled products, facilitating easy experimentation with different items.

"For Men" Products:

If products labeled "For Men" enhance your comfort, feel free to choose them. However, note that the distinction often lies in packaging. Don't hesitate to explore other aisles, as many products are unisex and suitable for all genders.

Exploration Strategies:

Subscription services provide a low-risk way to try new products. In physical stores, ask for samples before committing to full-sized purchases for a similar trial experience.

Shaving

Shaving stands as a fundamental aspect of a man's grooming routine, with the management of facial hair being a practice ingrained for thousands of years. As early as 300 B.C., Alexander the Great mandated his soldiers to maintain clean-shaven faces to prevent adversaries from seizing their beards in battle, initiating a lasting fixation on shaving.

The daily ritual of shaving may seem like a mundane task, and some men believe that growing a beard would require less upkeep. Spoiler alert: that's not the case, but more details on that later. Regardless of whether you opt for a clean-shaven look, a beard, or something in between, tending to your facial hair is inevitable. Rather than viewing it as a chore, integrate it into your self-care routine. Since you're already engaged in the practice, here's how to transform it into an experience you genuinely anticipate.

The Razor Dilemma

There's a fervent debate about the best razor, but the ideal one for you is the one that feels most comfortable on your skin. Shaving should not result in a face adorned with bandages.

Discovering a razor that provides a daily, minimally irritating experience involves some trial and error. To begin, familiarize yourself with the three main types of razors.

Multi-Blade Cartridge Razors:

Disposable cartridge razors are user-friendly, reasonably priced, and widely accessible. Nowadays, you can even have them delivered to your doorstep. Most feature multiple blades, believed to offer a closer shave. However, some argue that more blades increase the risk of ingrown hairs due to an overly close shave.

Single-Blade Safety Razors:

In recent years, the traditional single-blade safety razor has made a comeback. Advocates assert that these razors provide an excellent shave, particularly for sensitive skin, and help prevent razor bumps and ingrown hairs. They don't cut as close to the skin as multi-blade razors, making it easier for hair to regrow without snagging. The drawback is that the term "safety" is relative; they are prone to causing cuts and require some time to adapt to.

Electric Razor:

The primary appeal of an electric razor lies in its convenience. Most are designed for dry skin shaving, offering speed, portability, and simplicity. They might be suitable for individuals with sensitive skin as they can be gentler than traditional razors. However, they come with a cost and still require blade replacements at regular intervals.

How to Perform a Home Shave

Even if your dad didn't teach you, many guys admit they aren't quite sure how to shave properly.

Step 1: Open Pores
   Splash hot water on your face, use a hot towel, or take advantage of the shower to open pores and soften facial hair.

Step 2: Exfoliate Before Shaving
   Prevent blade clogging and nicks by exfoliating to remove dead skin cells. This also helps elevate hairs for a more effective shave.

Step 3: Apply Pre-Shave Oil
   Enhance razor glide by applying oil before shaving cream. This reduces the risk of razor burn caused by excessive pulling.

Step 4: Use Moisturizing Shaving Cream
   Opt for shaving cream with a rich lather and moisturizing ingredients to minimize post-shave irritation.

Step 5: Ensure a Sharp Blade
   Avoid cuts and razor burn by ensuring your razor is sharp; change cartridge razors after approximately three uses.

Step 6: Shave in the Direction of Hair Growth
   Follow the grain to prevent ingrown hairs and razor bumps.

Step 7: Rinse with Cold Water
   Calm your skin and close pores by rinsing off with cold water after shaving.

Step 8: Finish with Moisturizer

Seal the deal with post-shave lotion or moisturizer to soothe your skin, supporting its natural protective barrier.

<u>Why Opt for a Professional Barber Shave?</u>

Before Mr. King Gillette introduced the at-home disposable razor in 1895, men's sole option was to visit the barber. Committing to a barber shave required careful planning, as it typically took around an hour. When entrusting someone with a blade near your carotid artery, rushing was not an option.

In contemporary times, there may not be a necessity for a barber shave, but the experience is undeniably delightful. The unique sensation of a barber shave is unparalleled at home. Moreover, it serves as an excellent way to compel yourself to disconnect, even if only for a brief period. If considering a barber shave for a special occasion like a wedding, it's advisable to schedule it a day prior to allow for potential irritation. Better yet, indulge in one simply because—no special occasion required.

Wanna Keep the Beard
there's still upkeep to consider.
- Moisturize It: Prevent scraggly hair and dry skin beneath by massaging in moisturizer and using beard balm.
- Wash It: Regularly cleanse your beard with a dedicated beard wash to keep both hair and skin underneath clean.
- Trim It: Invest in an electric trimmer with adjustable length settings to maintain the beard shape, avoiding an unkempt appearance.

- Shape It: Visit a barber every three to four months to refine the beard lines and trim excess bulk.

- Shave (Some of) It: Maintain beard lines by shaving the neck, cheeks, and any areas with stray hairs.

When shopping for grooming products:

- Where to Go: Choose razors with easily accessible refills and explore shaving products from established men's skincare brands.

- How Much to Spend: Invest in a high-quality razor, considering online options for affordable refills, and save on supplementary items like shaving cream.

- How to Know If Something Is Good: Seek advice from friends with impressive beards, read online reviews, or consult your barber, who likely has ample shaving experience.

- Buy for Your Skin Type: Identify your skin type before purchasing shaving products, opting for sensitive skin or cooling ingredients like aloe if prone to breakouts or irritation. Men of color should choose brands formulated for their skin to reduce ingrown hairs.

- Cheaper Isn't Always Better: While avoiding excessive costs, prioritize products that make your skin feel good over selecting the lowest-priced options, as cheap razors may dull quickly and compromise the quality of the shave.

Masking

Masking has been a skincare staple for generations, and the popularity of sheet masks, fueled by the Korean skincare trend, has made them as common as deodorant. While you may have seen your female friends use them, if you haven't considered incorporating masks into your routine, you're overlooking a beneficial skincare practice.

Masks are particularly suited for men who prefer using minimal products and seek quicker results. These treatments are highly potent and focused, requiring less frequent application than other skincare items. While they don't replace a regular skincare routine, if daily care is likened to cardio, masking can be considered an interval workout.

Typically meant for use once a week or even less frequently, masks prove effective in addressing various skin concerns like breakouts, dryness, redness, and oiliness. Categorized into five main types, the choice depends on the specific results you're aiming for.

Clay Masks

When you think of a face mask, envision a sophisticated woman with cucumber slices on her eyes and a face coated in mud – the classic clay mask. Utilizing ingredients like mud, clay, and charcoal, these masks go beyond your regular cleanser, providing a deep clean to pores. As the mask dries, it acts like a vacuum, extracting dirt and grime from your pores, aiding in shine control and preventing breakouts.

How to Apply a Clay Mask

Begin by washing your face, leaving it slightly damp. Apply an even layer to your face, excluding the eyes and mouth. Allow it to dry for approximately 20 minutes; it may feel tight, which is normal. Rinse it off with warm water using your hands or a washcloth, and complete the routine with a moisturizer.

Peel-Off Masks

Similar to clay masks, peel-off masks aim to eliminate deep-seated pore buildup. They utilize adhesive substances known as polymers, which adhere to impurities and extract them upon mask removal. Effective for tackling blackheads and managing shine, but caution is needed as prolonged application may harm your skin barrier. Adhere strictly to the package instructions and avoid exceeding the recommended duration.

How to Apply a Peel-Off Mask

After washing and drying your face, apply a thin, uniform layer of the gel, excluding the eyes, mouth, eyebrows, and facial hair. Allow the gel to dry for the specified time on the bottle (typically 15–20 minutes), then gently peel it off. Use warm water to remove any residues and follow up with a moisturizer to reduce potential irritation.

Exfoliating Masks

Designed to eliminate dead skin cells on your skin's surface, exfoliating masks promote a brighter complexion and aid in reducing signs of aging. Unlike manual scrubs that require handwork, these masks employ acids to break the bonds between dead cells, requiring minimal effort and usage only once or twice a week.

How to Apply an Exfoliating Mask

While these masks are gentle, they contain acids, so it's important to read the instructions before the initial use and start with a clean face. Some masks should be left on for a specified time (typically around 20 minutes), while others are suitable for overnight wear. Regardless of the type, conclude with the application of a moisturizer.

Sheet Masks

The current resurgence in masking owes much to sheet masks, propelled into the limelight by social media. Not only do they appear amusing, but they also deliver tangible results. The concept is straightforward: these are one-time use, disposable masks typically crafted from serum-soaked paper. As the sheet rests on your face, it forms a barrier facilitating rapid absorption of the serum into your skin, preventing it from evaporating. With thousands of variations available, most sheet masks are gentle enough for daily use, although once or twice a week suffices.

How to Apply a Sheet Mask

Following face washing, open the package and unfold the mask, which features holes for your eyes, nose, and mouth. Align these with your face and smooth the mask down. Leave it on for approximately 15–30 minutes, then discard it. Gently pat any remaining serum into your skin.

Hydrating Masks

When your skin is exceptionally dry, especially during harsh winter or after a day at the beach, regular moisturizer might not suffice. In such cases, a hydrating mask becomes essential. Typically available in gel or cream forms, these masks contain ingredients like hyaluronic acid, aloe, and various botanical extracts. Unlike other masks, hydrating masks can be worn for extended periods and used more frequently, even on a daily basis for those with particularly dry or irritated skin.

How to Apply a Hydrating Mask

Following cleansing, generously apply the mask to your face, avoiding the eye area. Leave it on for the specified duration mentioned on the container. It may not completely dry, but when the time is up, rinse it off with warm water. Optionally, conclude with a moisturizer for added hydration.

Shopping List

Where to Shop: In this era of abundant masking options, you can find them almost anywhere, from your local grocery store to major retail outlets, and they are also easily accessible online.

Budget Consideration: Masks, especially sheet masks, tend to be affordable, posing minimal financial risk. Start with a reasonably priced option. If masking becomes a regular part of your routine, you might consider a slightly higher investment.

Quality Check: The surge in masking's popularity on social media offers a valuable starting point. Explore the masks you see people using on platforms like Instagram and give them a try. When making online purchases, always take the time to read reviews.

Opt for Multipacks: While individual sheet masks are budget-friendly, they offer only a single use. Consider opting for multipacks, which may have a higher initial cost but provide long-term savings.

Facials

Facials encompass a comprehensive self-care practice, combining relaxation with practical benefits that enhance your daily skincare routine. Just as a car runs more efficiently after a mechanic's check, facials, conducted by professionals, serve as a thorough inspection for your skin. While facials have often been overlooked in male grooming, they are now easily accessible, akin to getting a haircut. Experts recommend getting a facial at least four times a year, coinciding with seasonal changes that can impact your skin. Facials not only address immediate concerns, such as sweat-clogged pores from summer, but also provide valuable insights into your skincare routine's effectiveness. Consider professionals as the mechanics in this analogy, offering guidance for improvement. The self-esteem boost from walking out with a fresh, brighter face is an added bonus, making facials a compelling self-care investment. Don't hesitate – give your skin the reset it deserves.

What to Anticipate from a Facial

For those unfamiliar, facials may seem like an elaborate process easily replicable at home. However, the expertise of a professional adds value by identifying unseen issues, providing solutions to unexpected problems, and preemptively addressing potential future concerns. Before your initial facial experience, here's a breakdown of the process:

Step 1: Cleansing
Your aesthetician initiates the session with a thorough face cleansing, often performed twice to establish a clean canvas for subsequent steps.

Step 2: Inspection
Under a bright light, your skin undergoes careful examination, allowing the aesthetician to evaluate its condition and devise a customized plan.

Step 3: Exfoliation
Tailored to your skin's requirements, exfoliation methods such as enzyme peels, facial scrubs, or stronger options are employed, based on sensitivity and exfoliation needs.

Step 4: Extractions
Irrespective of breakout concerns, the aesthetician might recommend extractions. This involves skillfully removing debris and dirt from pores to prevent long-term marks. Extractions may involve mild discomfort, and the option to opt out is usually offered.

Step 5: Mask
Post-extractions, a soothing, hydrating serum and mask are applied to calm the skin, re-moisturize it, and minimize irritation.

Step 6: Treatments

Following the mask, additional serums and treatments are applied based on your skin's specific needs. Tools like oxygen or LED lights may be incorporated for enhanced results.

Step 7: Moisturizer/SPF

To conclude, the aesthetician prepares your skin for daily exposure by sealing in the benefits with moisturizer and applying SPF if the facial is conducted during daylight hours.

Where to Visit

The primary hurdle for most men in getting a facial often lies in stepping into a spa. Traditionally considered a luxury reserved for upscale spas, facials required the commitment of time, often involving sitting around in a robe – an inconvenience many men preferred to avoid. However, contemporary alternatives known as facial bars have emerged. These no-frills establishments focus exclusively on facials, offering a quick and easy experience without the need to change clothes. Ideal for maintenance, many even provide monthly memberships, seamlessly incorporating facials into your regular grooming routine.

When selecting a facial venue, prioritize your comfort. Consider the price, striking a balance between quality and affordability. Opt for a location that suits your convenience and aligns with the atmosphere you prefer – a place where you genuinely look forward to going. Establish a rapport with an aesthetician you feel comfortable seeing regularly; the more they familiarize themselves with your skin, the better equipped they are to assess and address potential issues proactively. Remember, you're not committed to one place; explore different options until you find the one that suits you best.

Teeth

It's straightforward: Happiness often translates into more smiles, showcasing your teeth—whether they're gleaming or not-so-pearly. Research indicates that the appearance of your teeth can significantly influence your self-esteem and overall mood. Notably, individuals facing depression may neglect their oral hygiene, while those content with their dental appearance tend to smile more, projecting an image of happiness and friendliness.

While oral hygiene is a crucial aspect of self-care with far-reaching effects, it tends to be overshadowed when discussing facial care. Let's change that perspective. Prioritizing good dental hygiene not only contributes to long-term health but also enhances happiness, potentially preserving a more youthful appearance.

Principles of Effective Dental Care

While many are familiar with the recommended dental care practices, adherence varies. Surveys indicate that only about 64% of American adults visit the dentist annually, and 23% have gone two or more days without brushing. Establishing a consistent oral hygiene routine is pivotal for long-term health and achieving an improved smile. Here's how to do it:

1. Brush Twice a Day: Following the American Dental Association (ADA) guidelines, everyone should brush their teeth for a full 2 minutes both in the morning and before bedtime, a frequency and duration often underestimated by the average person.

2. Use a Fluoride Toothpaste: Regardless of toothpaste preference, ensure it contains fluoride—a proven ingredient for strengthening teeth and preventing cavities. Even natural toothpaste should include fluoride for optimal dental health.

3. Floss after Brushing: Flossing immediately after brushing is proven to reduce decay, prevent cavities, and combat gum disease. Shockingly, only 40% of adults floss daily, emphasizing the importance of joining the majority who do. For those struggling with traditional flossing or sensitive gums, a water flosser is a viable alternative.

4. Utilize an Alcohol-Free Mouth Rinse: While not universally endorsed, incorporating a mouthwash into your routine can help eliminate oral bacteria and combat bad breath. Opt for alcohol-free formulas to avoid potential drying effects.

5. Consider Tongue Scraping: Although less popular in Western cultures, Ayurvedic medicine advocates daily tongue scraping for enhanced dental hygiene. Adopting this practice can be a unique way to elevate your oral care routine.

The Choice of Your Toothbrush Matters

The effectiveness of your oral hygiene is closely tied to the tools you select, with the toothbrush being the most crucial in your arsenal. According to the ADA, both manual and electric toothbrushes can be efficient if used for the recommended 2 minutes, twice a day. Recognizing the likelihood of the average person falling short of this, dentists often suggest electric toothbrushes to eliminate plaque and bacteria with minimal effort and reduced user error.

An electric toothbrush brings advantages by removing guess-work. Many come equipped with automatic timers that shut off after the recommended 2 minutes, and they excel in breaking up plaque, especially in challenging areas like between teeth, more efficiently than manual toothbrushes. Some models even prompt you to change the brush head every three to four months. However, it's worth noting that these toothbrushes can be pricey. If it fits your budget, an upgrade is worthwhile, but if not, the best toothbrush for you is the one you'll consistently use.

At-Home Teeth Whitening

A desire for a brighter smile is common, as white teeth not only signify good health but also contribute to a more youthful and vibrant appearance. While daily dental care aids in maintaining whiteness by eliminating surface stains, many seek additional methods. At-home whitening products have gained popularity for this reason, and here are some prevalent ways to enhance your smile:

1. Whitening Toothpaste: These toothpaste variants contain small abrasive elements that physically remove stains during brushing. Dentists caution against daily use due to potential enamel weakening. Alternatively, consider whitening toothpaste with hydrogen peroxide or apple cider vinegar to aid stain removal.

2. Stick-On Strips: Coated in a bleaching agent, these strips adhere to your teeth for a designated time, effectively and safely lightening tooth color with consistent use. Dentists appreciate their mildness and gentleness when used correctly.

3. LED Light Therapy: A recent trend in teeth whitening involves LED light therapy paired with bleaching gels. The light enhances the effectiveness of the bleach, facilitating deeper penetration. Additionally, it is considered gentler on sensitive teeth and gums.

4. Whitening Pen: These products serve as targeted treatments for specific teeth, akin to markers. The paintbrush-like tip is saturated with a bleaching agent, allowing direct application to address specific stains. Ideal for travel or addressing isolated concerns.

Anti-Aging

The notion that men age like fine wines, described as rugged and distinguished, implies a positive transformation over time. However, there's a delicate balance between appearing mature and looking old, and no one wishes to cross that line.

While it may seem acceptable for men to lack a robust anti-aging routine, this perception becomes problematic when aging signs become more apparent. Men often neglect self-care and address aging concerns belatedly. The key insight into anti-aging is the necessity to start early. While there's no magic product to completely erase wrinkles, a well-rounded skincare routine with suitable ingredients can decelerate their onset, preventing a sudden resemblance to a raisin.

In contrast to women, who are taught early on to proactively combat aging, men need to adopt a similar proactive mindset rather than reacting later in life. Acknowledging that men worry about aging as much as women, despite not openly discussing it, is crucial in preparing for the aging process.

As individuals age, the skin experiences a gradual decline in collagen production, leading to reduced tightness. Additionally, facial fat decreases, contributing to wrinkles and sagging skin. In men, signs typically manifest around the eyes, chin, and neck, with forehead lines and brow furrows appearing over time. Dryness and redness may also become more prominent.

Aging isn't something to fear; it's a natural aspect of life. Self-care involves meeting your needs, and addressing signs of aging can be one of the benefits if that aligns with your goals. An anti-aging-focused skincare routine goes beyond trying to halt aging; it enhances overall skin appearance. Establishing a sustainable daily skincare routine is the foundation, followed by incorporating additional measures for comprehensive care.

Exfoliation

You're likely familiar with the concept and importance of exfoliation, but its significance becomes more pronounced with age. Aging slows down the natural regeneration of skin cells, extending the average turnover period to approximately twenty-eight days. Consequently, as you age, dead skin cells linger on the skin's surface, leading to issues like dryness, rough patches, and an uneven skin tone. Additionally, aging may make your skin more sensitive, potentially rendering your usual facial scrub too abrasive. Instead, opt for a chemical exfoliant regularly, seeking products with alpha hydroxy acids such as glycolic or lactic acid, along with beta hydroxy acids like salicylic acid. These acids delicately dissolve the bonds attaching dead skin cells without the need for physical scrubbing. While some products are gentle enough for daily use, if you're new to chemical exfoliants, start with once or twice a week and gradually increase frequency.

Hydrate

Hydrating stands as the fundamental step in any skincare regimen, growing even more crucial with age. The aging process not only diminishes the skin's collagen production but also reduces its capacity to maintain moisture. Dry skin, as a result, appears lackluster, thinner, and more prone to fine lines and wrinkles. Consistent use of moisturizer is essential, especially as you age, and you may find it necessary to shift to heavier creams that deeply hydrate and lock in moisture. Seek products featuring hyaluronic acid, a natural substance aiding water retention in cells, and ceramides, which create a protective layer to prevent moisture loss.

Vitamin C

The skin's aging signs are linked to free radicals, triggered by factors like sun exposure, environmental pollution, and diet, causing damage to healthy cells by electron theft. The most effective defense against free radicals is antioxidants, with vitamin C reigning supreme. Just as vitamin C strengthens the immune system internally, it proves beneficial for the skin when incorporated into skincare products. Vitamin C counteracts oxidative stress from free radicals, contributing to brighter skin, a more even tone, lightening of sun spots and hyperpigmentation, and even preventing the deepening of lines and wrinkles. To harness its benefits, integrate a vitamin C serum into your routine, applying it after cleansing and before moisturizing.

Retinol

Dermatologists emphasize the significance of incorporating retinol into your skincare, whether aging is a concern or not. This form of vitamin A, extensively studied for decades, proves effective in addressing various issues, from aging to acne, and potentially preventing certain skin cancers. The key lies in its mechanism: Retinol operates beneath the skin surface, fostering cell turnover and maintaining the proper regenerative cycle. As skin cell renewal tends to slow with age, retinol helps counteract this process. If acne has been a concern, you might already be using it as the active ingredient in many prescription acne products. If not, consider incorporating it gradually, starting with once a week at night after cleansing, and gradually increasing frequency. Due to potential skin irritation, especially initially, be cautious and apply it exclusively at night. Additionally, as retinol can heighten skin sensitivity to the sun, it's essential to wear sunscreen during the day.

Sunscreen

The consensus among dermatologists is that sunscreen serves not only as a preventive measure against skin cancer but also stands as one of the most potent anti-aging solutions. UV ray-induced damage has been associated with various aging signs, including wrinkles and sagging skin, primarily due to the free radicals generated by sun exposure, causing cellular havoc. Sunscreen emerges as the optimal defense against these effects and should be incorporated into your daily routine. If you haven't embraced this practice yet, now is the time to start.

Part 4: Hair Care

Regardless of your hair type or volume, everyone desires fantastic hair, as it is an integral aspect of the human experience. Whether we like it or not, our hair conveys a lot about us, a tradition observed throughout history (cue Samson) with humans dedicating substantial time to styling, cutting, coloring, and maintaining it.

Research indicates that one's perception of their hair significantly influences their mood. The "Good Hair Day Effect" illustrates that when you believe your hair looks good—perhaps right after a salon visit or when you've expertly styled it—your posture improves, you smile more, exhibit friendliness, and experience increased confidence. This universal experience occurs when you catch your reflection and think, "Wow, I look great."

This very phenomenon underscores why hair care falls within the realm of self-care. It transcends mere external aesthetics or maintaining hair health; it's about how your hair influences your internal well-being and can positively impact your life. As self-care emphasizes, if an activity doesn't contribute to feeling good, why engage in it?

Ditch the All-in-One

Achieving a fantastic hairstyle begins with proper hair care. Many men view hair care as a quick task to check off during their shower routine. This is why multiuse products gained popularity, with the belief that consolidating hair products would encourage men to use them.

However, a revelation is in order: Products designed for body washing are not suitable for your hair. Opting for the right hair care products not only enhances the appearance and manageability of your hair but may also contribute to maintaining its health in the long run. Consider caring for your hair as not only an enhancement for what's on your head but also a positive influence on your overall life. It all commences with your shower routine.

Hair Care Tips

Taking care of your hair involves more than just ensuring it's clean; it's about promoting both better appearance and overall health. Follow these tips for optimal hair care:

1. Avoid Multiuse Products: While shampoo/conditioner combos sound convenient, they often fall short in delivering specialized care. Opt for separate shampoos and conditioners or a cleansing conditioner for curly hair.

2. Limit Shampooing: Washing your hair daily can lead to dryness. Aim for every other day or longer intervals, especially if your hair is short. Consider sulfate-free shampoos to retain natural oils.

3. Choose the Right Shampoo: Tailor your shampoo choice to your hair type. Volumizing shampoos add body to thin hair, while moisturizing shampoos cater to the needs of curly hair.

4. Always Use Conditioner: Replenish lost moisture by using conditioner with every shampoo, even for short hair. Longer hair requires more attention as it tends to dry out faster.

5. Scalp Massage: Prioritize scalp health by gently massaging your scalp with your fingertips and nails during shampooing. This promotes blood flow and helps remove dead skin.

6. Incorporate a Scalp Scrub: Treat your scalp like a garden, clearing debris with a scalp scrub about once a week. Ensure it doubles as a shampoo or use it before your regular shampoo.

7. Gentle Drying: Treat wet hair delicately, whether thinning or not. Pat your hair dry with a towel instead of rubbing to minimize breakage and preserve natural texture.

Understanding Shampoo Labels

Among personal grooming products, shampoo bottles often feature perplexing terminology. Here's a breakdown of these terms:

1. Sulfate-Free: Sulfates are chemicals that create lather in cleansing products. While people expect lather from soap, sulfates are thought to excessively strip oil from hair. Many experts now recommend sulfate-free shampoo.

2. Paraben-Free: Preservatives are essential for grooming products to remain shelf-stable. Parabens, traditional preservatives, have faced scrutiny for potential cancer links, though conclusive medical evidence is lacking.

3. Phthalate-Free: These chemicals contribute to gel textures and prolonged artificial fragrance in grooming products. Considered endocrine disruptors, they may be associated with certain cancers.

4. Silicone-Free: Silicone provides a smooth feeling in grooming products, creating a protective coating on hair. Advocates claim it prevents damage, while critics argue it may suffocate hair, causing more harm than good.

5. Anti-Dandruff: Dandruff stems from a scalp fungus, and true anti-dandruff shampoos include antifungal ingredients like zinc pyrithione and ketoconazole. Effective against dandruff, they may not address issues caused by different factors. Consult your dermatologist before switching to dandruff shampoo.

Hairdryer

In the iconic Saturday Night Fever movie, John Travolta's character, Tony Manero, prepares to go out, placing significant emphasis on styling his hair, notably using a blow dryer to achieve a voluminous look. This enduring grooming moment underscores the importance of a blow dryer in shaping hair, enhancing product efficacy, and expediting the drying process. Your barber or hairstylist recognizes this, utilizing a blow dryer to perfect your haircut. It's a crucial tool in their arsenal and should be in yours too. Regardless of hair length, a blow dryer can be a game-changer. If you haven't embraced this tool, consider trying one at the gym before investing in an affordable option for home use. While high-end dryers exist, a basic version works well for most unless you're a professional stylist or aiming for intricate styles. Unsure how to use it? Here's what you need to know.

Hair dryers typically consist of standard elements, regardless of their cost. While pricier options offer additional features, whether you utilize them is a personal choice.

1. Heat Setting: Most hair dryers feature low, medium, and high heat settings, allowing control over the heat applied to

your hair and scalp.

2. Fan Setting: Multiple fan settings regulate the speed of the airflow. While not as crucial as heat settings, sticking to medium or low prevents potential frizz caused by high settings.

3. Concentrator: This attachment, resembling an end cap with a slit, concentrates air through a smaller area, facilitating precise targeting. Valuable for styles like pompadours that require front volume.

4. Diffuser: Less common than concentrators, a diffuser disperses air across a broader area, ideal for curly hair, preserving natural texture without inducing frizz during rapid drying.

5. Cold Button: Included in most dryers, the cold button turns off the heater, allowing cold air to set the style once hair is dry.

Using a Hair Dryer:

Step 1: Comb Out Tangles
While hair is damp, comb through to eliminate tangles, shaping it into the desired style.

Step 2: Apply Product to Wet Hair
For certain products like gels and water-based pomades, apply a small amount to damp hair, shaping it as the blow dryer activates the product.

Step 3: Don't Hold It Too Close to Your Head
Maintain a 6 to 8-inch distance between the hair dryer and

your head to prevent potential scalp burns.

Step 4: Use It to Direct the Hair

Employ the hair dryer to shape your hair as it dries. Point the nozzle in the desired direction for styling.

Step 5: Use a Brush

While directing the air, use a brush to keep your hair in place, ensuring roots dry quickly for enhanced volume.

Step 6: Don't Overuse It

Avoid excessive use to prevent heat damage. Once your hair is dried to your liking, turn off the dryer to avoid counterproductive over-drying.

Enhance your hair drying experience with these advanced tips:

1. Utilize the Cold Setting: The cold setting serves a purpose beyond cooling down. After using heat to make your hair malleable, switch to the cold setting once it's dry. This blasts cool air, locking your style in place for longer-lasting results.

2. High Heat Isn't Always Necessary: Contrary to the belief that more heat is better, it's not always the case. Opt for the medium setting for most hair types, reserving high heat for healthier hair. If your hair is fine or thin, the low setting helps preserve and add volume.

3. Dry Underneath by Flipping Your Head: For those with longer hair, flip your head upside down during drying. This

technique not only ensures the underside is dry but also adds volume, preventing a flat appearance.

4. Finger Styling for Texture: When aiming for a messy, textured look, use your fingers instead of a brush. While brushes provide a polished finish, fingers offer a messier yet controlled result, perfect for achieving that textured appearance.

Hair Products

Taking care of your hair is the initial step towards achieving an impressive mane, but it doesn't end there. Styling plays a crucial role, and while styling products can be beneficial, their vast variety can be bewildering. Understanding their functions is one aspect, while knowing how to apply them is another.

According to professional hairstylists, a common error among men is using excessive amounts of styling products. Another mistake is using these products to forcefully control the hair. The intended purpose of styling products is to enhance your natural hair without completely transforming its appearance.

Let's be honest: Your primary concern is how your hair looks. This is why styling your hair is a vital act of self-care, just like ensuring its overall health. Consider these products as tools to optimize your hair's appearance, similar to wearing a well-fitted suit. Here's a guide on how to make the most of them.

Varieties of Hair Products

The selection of the appropriate hair product hinges on your desired outcome and your specific hair type.

1. Pomade: Initially oil-based, it's now predominantly water-based and is available in numerous variations. Versatile and well-suited for most men's hair, it excels in parting and slicking. Matte versions are ideal for a more casual appearance.

2. Clay: Similar to pomade but without shine, it provides a dry, natural finish. It enhances separation, texture, and suits messy hairstyles.

3. Wax: Typically wax-based, heavy, shiny, and, well, waxy. It offers more shine than pomade, providing substantial control. Ideal for shaping coarse, textured hair by locking in moisture without compromising hold.

4. Paste: Creamier than pomade, with less hold and added moisture, making it perfect for curly or wavy hair. Leaves a natural, non-shiny finish, suitable for longer styles needing texture.

5. Gel: Traditionally associated with high shine and immovable hairstyles, modern gels are lighter. As it dries, it forms a coating on the hair, maintaining the styled shape. Also used to define curls and protect against frizz.

6. Cream: Resembling lotion, it hydrates and suits curly or wavy hair but is versatile for any hair type. Smoothes hair, retains natural texture, and provides hold for a natural appearance.

7. Salt Spray: A contemporary version of the old mix of table salt and water. Contains healthy oils and natural salt for texture

without overdrying. Ideal for a piecey surfer look and adds volume without greasiness, making it suitable for thinning hair.

8. Hair Spray: Secures your style and offers protection throughout the day. Modern versions provide strong hold without excessive stiffness. Forms a protective barrier against various elements, starting with a light application to prevent overly rigid styles.

Using Hair Products Effectively

Consult any hairstylist, and they'll inform you that many men misuse hair products. Here's how to avoid being one of those individuals.

1. Begin with Damp Hair: Most contemporary products are water-soluble, making them easier to apply on damp hair. Unless specified otherwise, apply onto towel-dried hair and then use a hair dryer.

2. Optimal Quantity: Regardless of the product, start with a pea- to dime-sized amount. You can add more if needed, but putting in too much may require a return to the shower.

3. Cover Your Hands: Ensure your entire palms are covered by rubbing the product between your hands. Work the product between your fingers, which will be used for shaping your hair.

4. Commence at the Back: Start applying the product at the back of your hair and move forward. Initiating from the back ensures a more uniform application, and you can add more in

the front if necessary.

5. Thorough Distribution, Then Shaping: While applying, ensure thorough distribution throughout your hair. Once massaged in, go back and shape your hair into the desired style.

6. Hair Spray as the Final Step: Once your style is completely dry, secure it with hairspray. Apply it directly to your hair (lightly) or spray it onto a brush and run it through your hair.

Shopping Guide

Where to Shop: Begin at the place where you purchase your shampoo or grooming items. If you already have a preferred shampoo brand, check if they also offer styling products. When shopping online, pay attention to suggested similar products based on your purchases.

Budget Considerations: Higher prices don't always equate to better performance. Don't fixate too much on costs. If you're trying something new, opt for an affordable version initially to gauge your preferences and results.

Assessing Product Quality: Most hair products look similar on the shelf, making it challenging to determine suitability. The best way to find the right one for you is to experiment. This may involve some time and expenditure. Start with a cost-effective option and be open to trying a few.

Seek Advice: Consult your barber for recommendations; they

have extensive experience and insights. Additionally, inquire with friends who maintain great hair or explore the products favored by a celebrity with enviable locks—online resources often feature articles where celebrities or their stylists discuss their preferred products.

Barbers & Hair stylists

The barber holds a significant role in a man's life, whether it's a long-standing relationship or changing barbers as frequently as clothes. This person, entrusted with cutting your hair, wields considerable influence, fostering connections based on trust, communication, and often friendship. Barbershops, in some communities, serve as unofficial gathering spots and social centers. Some clients prefer a silent experience in the barber's chair, and that's perfectly acceptable.

Choosing who cuts your hair extends beyond the literal act, influencing your overall well-being. When you look good, you feel good, and barbers or hairstylists aim for their clients to leave feeling amazing. Consider them as guides in your self-care journey; self-care is about feeling good, and it doesn't always have to be a solitary effort.

Deciding who cuts your hair is a personal choice, involving more than just the haircut itself. Recognizing the distinctions between barbers and hairstylists is crucial in making an informed decision. Their roles and the experiences they offer differ, and understanding these differences empowers you to make the most out of your choice. Ultimately, the decision rests with you, but being informed is key to optimizing the experience.

Barbers:

Traditionally, barbers were trained not only in hair cutting but also in shaving and beard trimming, contributing to the perception that barbers are for men, while stylists are for women. However, contemporary barberships often blur these gender-based distinctions. While modern barbers still provide shaves and beard trims, their primary focus is on shorter, more traditional men's haircuts using clippers. The barber experience is straightforward, typically omitting hair washing before cutting, eschewing services like color, and emphasizing efficiency.

Reasons to Choose a Barber:
  1. No-fuss experience with walk-ins and quick appointments.
  2. Generally more affordable, although upscale barbershops are changing this.
  3. Ideal for simple haircuts like crew cuts or fades.

Reasons Not to Choose a Barber:
  1. For longer hair or styles requiring more styling, consider a hairstylist.
  2. If you seek services beyond a basic haircut, such as color.

Hairstylists:

The distinction between a hairstylist and a barber is rooted in training. Hairstylists acquire cosmetology licenses, attending cosmetology school to learn not only cutting and styling but also color, perms, and manicures. They typically use scissors more frequently than clippers due to their diverse training. Hairstylists invest more time in learning to cut women's hair, adapting their approach for men as needed.

Reasons to Choose a Hairstylist:

1. Suitable for longer cuts or styles requiring additional styling.

2. Some argue that cuts from hairstylists grow out better, potentially requiring less frequent visits.

3. Capable of services like hair coloring or other treatments.

4. Typically includes hair washing before cutting.

Reasons Not to Choose a Hairstylist:

1. Tends to be pricier than barbers, with longer appointment durations.

2. If you're seeking a quick appointment or a simple haircut like a buzz, a barber might be a better choice.

Determining an Appropriate Haircut Cost

While the expense of a haircut often influences your choice of salon, it should not be the sole consideration. Opting for the cheapest option may not be the best strategy. The quality of a haircut is noticeable, revealing itself in the details. A hastily and bluntly cut hair may not look appealing as it grows out, and poorly executed elements like an uneven neck fade indicate a budget haircut.

This doesn't imply that you need to allocate a substantial amount each month for your hair. Instead, conduct thorough research. Seek recommendations from friends with impressive hairstyles, read reviews of local establishments, or explore Instagram for barbershops and salons in your vicinity. Once you've identified appealing options, review their prices online. Select a place with a price that aligns with your comfort level. After trying it out, if you're satisfied with the haircut, you've found your new spot. If not, move on to the next one on your list.

How to Approach Getting a Haircut

Whether you've been loyal to the same place for years or are exploring new options, there are established guidelines to enhance your haircut experience.

1. Establish a Routine:
   - Aim for a haircut every four to six weeks to maintain a polished appearance, avoiding unkempt neck and sideburns.

2. Utilize Visuals:
   - When contemplating a new style or visiting a new barber, bring pictures for reference. Select images featuring hairstyles you desire and be ready to convey what aspects you appreciate.

3. Visuals Over Verbal Descriptions:
   - Avoid using barber terms heard from others (such as fade or undercut) and rely on visuals to avoid miscommunication. Many barbers note that clients often misuse these terms.

4. Inquire about Styling:

- Prior to the haircut, discuss styling techniques with your barber. If you're not willing to invest time in styling, it's crucial to align expectations for a satisfactory result.

5. Acknowledge Their Expertise:

- Trust your barber's expertise. If they suggest a particular cut might not suit you, remain open-minded. Barbers possess professional insights into your hair and face shape that you might not be aware of. Engage in open communication and value their advice.

Hair loss

While we've extensively discussed hair care, a primary concern for many men is retaining their hair. Hair loss and thinning affect nearly every guy, and you're likely no exception.

This concern is not mere perception. Hair loss impacts men universally, transcending age. According to the American Hair Loss Association, two-thirds of men experience hair loss by age thirty-five, rising to 85 percent as they age. Experts often encounter patients expressing hair loss concerns in their early to mid-twenties, sometimes as early as late teens.

The psychological impact of losing hair is profound, affecting self-esteem, relationships, sexuality, and motivation. Many perceive it as a diminishing symbol of masculinity or attractiveness, making self-care challenging.

Genetics largely contribute to hair loss, and it's beyond your control. However, early intervention is crucial. If you anticipate hair loss, especially if it's a family pattern, take proactive measures to slow the process. While you can't regrow lost hair, you can preserve what remains.

Consulting a professional is the first step, followed by comprehending the situation and experimenting with treatments to find a suitable approach. Patience is essential, as both hair loss and its treatment are gradual processes. Experts suggest waiting three to six months to observe results after initiating treatment. When all else fails, there's no shame in opting for a short haircut as a practical solution.

Understanding Hair Loss Causes

The predominant form of hair loss in men is androgenetic alopecia, commonly known as male pattern baldness (MPB). This genetic condition is often associated with X chromosomes from the mother's side, but recent research indicates a contribution from the father's side as well. Recognizable signs of MPB include a receding hairline, a bald spot on the crown, and thinning on the top of the head. While MPB is genetic and challenging to prevent, it can be managed.

However, MPB is not the sole cause of hair loss; it can also be linked to internal diseases, inadequate diet, prescription medications, and lifestyle choices. Hair loss in areas beyond the hairline or crown may suggest a different cause, necessitating consultation with a physician or hair loss expert before initiating treatment.

The mechanism behind hair loss involves the male sex hormone dihydrotestosterone (DHT) and the enzyme 5-alpha-reductase, which converts testosterone to DHT. Genetic factors causing MPB upset this balance, resulting in elevated DHT levels in the scalp. Increased DHT prompts certain hair follicles to shrink, go dormant, and eventually die.

The hair growth cycle comprises three phases: growth, intermediate, and shedding. In scalps with elevated DHT levels, the growth and intermediate phases shorten, while the shedding phase prolongs, leading to thinning and loss.

Regarding a cure, once a hair follicle dies, it cannot be revived. However, distinguishing between completely dead and dormant follicles is challenging. Treatment may still yield improvements, especially if hair loss is not solely due to MPB. A doctor can create a personalized treatment plan based on individual needs.

To address hair loss, consulting a doctor is crucial to ensure appropriate treatment timing. Over-the-counter products like finasteride and minoxidil regulate DHT both externally and internally. Scalp care, including scrubs and serums, is essential to foster an optimal environment for hair growth. Natural remedies involving botanicals such as ginseng and technological advances like platelet-rich plasma (PRP) injections, derived from the patient's blood, offer promising options for regrowth. Always consult with an expert before attempting any treatment.

Impact of Lifestyle Choices on Hair Health

Transforming your hair isn't just about altering your products; subtle shifts in lifestyle can significantly influence your hair.

1. Prioritize Sleep:
   - Insufficient high-quality sleep disrupts the body's regen-

erative functions, potentially leading to various health issues, including hair loss.

2. Improve Diet:
  - Essential for hair growth, protein and biotin are crucial ingredients. Inadequate consumption of these elements can hinder proper hair growth. Additionally, incorporating fatty acids, antioxidants, and zinc into your diet supports healthy hair growth.

3. Manage Stress:
  - Elevated stress levels can induce follicles into a dormant state or trigger the immune system to attack them. Taking a holistic approach to combat hair loss often involves stress reduction as a primary goal.

4. Exercise Wisely:
  - While exercise is beneficial for overall health, excessive physical activity has been associated with temporary hair loss in some studies. If you engage in rigorous exercise, ensure a balanced intake of vitamins and proteins to counteract potential effects.

Part 5: Personal Space

Your residence, regardless of the time spent within, holds significant importance in your life. While it should undoubtedly mirror your taste and style, its paramount role is to be a place where you feel at ease. Many of the self-care practices discussed in this book can be carried out at home, a vital component of a robust self-care routine. However, if your home lacks the comfort you desire, it becomes challenging to unwind and concentrate on self-care. Creating a relaxing atmosphere at home is essential, as a serene home environment is the foundation for an effective self-care routine.

While the idea of living in a spacious mansion with dedicated areas for self-care activities, like a private gym or meditation room, may be appealing, it's not a necessity for cultivating a successful self-care routine. For many individuals, such luxuries are not realistic. The reassuring news is that it doesn't matter! Regardless of its size, any home can be optimized for self-care. With minimal effort, strategic adjustments, and perhaps the addition of a few houseplants or scented candles, your dwelling can transform into a self-care sanctuary akin to a spa.

TRANSFORMING YOUR HOME FOR SELF-CARE EXCELLENCE

Elevating your home for optimal self-care merely requires a shift in perspective. Initiating the process by creating versatile spaces is a smart approach. When space is limited, reconsider the setup, envisioning the various activities possible (such as transforming a reading nook into a meditation and yoga area). Instead of fitting your self-care routine into your home, organize your living space around your self-care regimen.

Maintaining cleanliness is equally crucial. You don't need to watch Marie Kondo on Netflix to recognize that clutter induces stress. Creating a comfortable space doesn't mean endorsing hoarding. Psychologically, clutter absorbs negative energy, while physically, it impedes airflow and hinders breathing. Crafting a welcoming and positive space is a personal journey. Surround yourself with elements that bring joy and promote relaxation. Remember, your home should serve as a sanctuary for rest and rejuvenation. To enhance each room, follow these steps systematically.

Living Room

Commence with the room you inhabit most frequently, likely the living room.

Emphasize Fundamental Seating

The cornerstone of the living room lies in seating, often centered around the couch. Opt for a proportionate couch that harmonizes with the room's dimensions, avoiding overpowering it. If space constraints dictate a smaller couch, complement it with a couple of accent chairs that not only align visually but also offer equal comfort.

Deemphasize the TV as the Focal Point

Rather than orienting the room around the TV, consider mounting it on the wall or situating it in a corner. This strategy fosters a tranquil ambiance conducive to relaxation and unhindered conversation with guests, devoid of the TV dominating the setting.

Establish Optimal Lighting

Swap out harsh overhead lighting for softer fixtures with multiple bulbs, dispersing light evenly. Incorporate accent lamps to reduce reliance on the overhead fixture. Installing dimmers on light switches is a simple upgrade, allowing personalized control over lighting.

Rugs Instead of Carpet

Opt for hardwood floors instead of wall-to-wall carpeting, as they are easier to clean and promote better airflow. Introduce stylish accent rugs strategically around the room, beneath the coffee table or chairs, providing floor protection and sound muffling.

Integrate Genuine Art

Enhance the homely ambiance with art, steering clear of commonplace movie posters or record sleeves. Art need not be expensive; consider high-quality printouts of appealing online photos, unique pieces from rummage sales, or budget-friendly original prints from platforms like Etsy. Utilize online framing services for cost-effective framing solutions.

<u>Kitchen</u>

Cultivate a kitchen that beckons you, encouraging more time spent cooking.

Organize Tools and Ingredients

Ensure food and kitchen tools are organized for easy access and efficient cleaning. Invest in a spice rack to eliminate constant cabinet digging, and store loose items like flour or nuts in clear glass containers for both aesthetic appeal and easy visibility.

Maintain Fridge Hygiene

Regularly wipe down fridge shelves and drawers to enhance visual appeal and prolong food freshness. Discard old or expired items promptly. Place an open box of baking soda inside to absorb odors. Remember to clean the exterior during interior cleaning sessions.

Essential Kitchen Tools

Facilitate cooking by investing in basic kitchen tools such as pots, pans, spatulas, knives, and cutting boards. Having the right tools enhances the ease and speed of cooking. For guidance on usage, explore curated kitchen kits or watch instructional videos on platforms like YouTube.

Elevate Dish Soap Experience

Transform your kitchen experience by opting for a dish soap with a different scent. Citrus scents energize, while floral scents like lavender offer a calming effect. The change in scent can make dishwashing less tedious, leaving a pleasant lingering aroma in the kitchen.

Incorporate a Table

Even in a compact space, introducing a small table and a few chairs transforms the kitchen's ambiance. It provides an alternative dining space beyond the couch or TV, inviting others into the room while you cook, turning the potentially isolating experience into a shared one.

Bedroom

Considering the average person spends one-third of their life sleeping, optimize the bedroom for restful sleep.

Enhance Pillow Collection

Multiple pillows not only enhance shared sleeping arrangements but can also contribute to a more restful sleep. Experiment with pillows of varying softness to discover the ideal combination for optimal sleep quality.

Invest in Quality Sheets

Quality sheets significantly impact sleep quality. Focus on material rather than thread count; linen sheets offer breathability, while flannel sheets provide warmth in colder seasons. Prioritize the tactile feel by testing sheets or taking advantage of trial offers, ensuring a texture that aligns with your preferences. Always include matching pillowcases.

Incorporate a Bedside Table

Allocate space for a bedside table, providing accessibility to items like an alarm clock or a book. This contributes to a relaxing environment, facilitating bedtime routines outlined in Part 2.

Maintain Clothing Order

Prevent bedroom clutter by investing in a hamper and

utilizing it consistently. Position it in a corner or within the closet, emphasizing the importance of placing dirty clothes inside rather than on the floor or bed. This practice prevents odor retention and supports optimal airflow in the bedroom, where air quality holds paramount significance.

Dual Light Control

Acknowledge the significance of light for sleep and ensure ample natural light enters the bedroom. Install blinds to regulate light filtration and invest in curtains for light blockage during challenging sleep periods.

HOW TO TRANSFORM YOUR BATHROOM INTO A SELF-CARE HAVEN

You might be questioning the need for an entire section dedicated to the bathroom, but let's face it—when it comes to implementing the various practices discussed in this book, the bathroom takes center stage. Your bathroom serves as the epicenter of self-care. Unless you're resorting to bathing in the kitchen sink or cleansing your face with an outdoor hose, your self-care routine inherently involves spending time in the bathroom.

While self-care should be a desire, an unwelcoming bathroom environment can diminish the likelihood of dedicating time to it. Overcoming the obstacles to self-care may require a shift in perspective, starting with how you perceive your surroundings.

A simple and effective approach involves giving your bathroom a self-care-centric facelift. This doesn't entail wielding a sledgehammer for a dramatic HGTV-style transformation. Instead, it involves a fresh perspective. Rather than viewing the bathroom merely as a functional necessity or a space to hastily navigate, envision it as a sanctuary. While the notion of a "spa atmosphere" in the bathroom may elicit a chuckle, those expressing such desires on House Hunters are onto something significant. In the realm of self-care, your bathroom should consistently be a space you genuinely want to inhabit.

<u>Transforming Your Bathroom into Your Preferred Space</u>

Irrespective of your bathroom's size or the number of individuals sharing it, with the right setup, any bathroom can evolve into a self-care haven. Follow these steps, and you'll find it hard to step away.

1. Embrace Simplicity: Regardless of your home's overall aesthetic, simplicity is key in the bathroom. Excessive decor and clutter shrink any room, and given that bathrooms tend to be the smallest, opt for light, neutral colors to create a brighter and more open feel.

2. Efficient Storage: Whether your product collection is extensive or minimal, maintain organization. Utilize shower caddies or shelving units to keep items off the floor and sides of the tub. Swap a standalone mirror for a medicine cabinet to keep products accessible yet out of sight. Open shelves offer additional storage without hindering airflow.

3. Considered Lighting: Just as overhead lighting may not suffice in other parts of your home, the same applies to the bathroom. Explore options like a lighted mirror to counteract unflattering overhead light. Install sconces or alternate lighting

sources for versatility, and a dimmer switch is particularly useful for creating a soothing ambiance during bath time.

4. Convenient Supplies: Organize your bathroom shelves, ensuring frequently used products are easily accessible. This applies to your self-care essentials. Keep bath supplies like oils and salts in a designated spot within the bathroom for easy access when preparing to unwind.

5. Introduce Greenery: Certain plant varieties, especially those from tropical climates, thrive in high-humidity bathrooms. Place potted plants on shelves or windowsills to enliven the space and enhance air quality.

6. Adapt to Showers: Even without a bathtub, a bathroom can be transformed into a self-care retreat. Invest in a shower stool for aromatherapy and relaxation benefits while the water is running, mimicking the experience of a bath.

<u>Transformative Elements</u>

When direct alterations to your bathroom space have limitations, there are game-changing products and adjustments that can deliver a similar impact.

1. Upgrade Your Towels:
   Opting for plush, soft towels in coordinating solid colors, akin to upgrading your sheets, is a minor change with substantial benefits. While larger towels are generally preferred, it's crucial to distinguish between beach towels and those intended for bathroom use.

2. Luxurious Hand Soap:

Elevating your hand soap from the standard to a more luxurious version is a simple upgrade that induces a remarkable sense of well-being. Choose hand soaps with natural ingredients and essential oils, ensuring a pleasant fragrance that lingers in the air post-wash.

3. Essential Oil Diffuser:

Beyond self-care, bathrooms fulfill practical purposes. Rather than resorting to air fresheners or matches, introduce an essential oil diffuser to consistently imbue the air with a delightful scent. This not only accelerates the dissipation of unpleasant odors but also maintains a refreshing atmosphere.

4. Thoughtful Shower Curtain:

As the unavoidable focal point in many bathrooms, the shower curtain can significantly influence the overall aesthetic. Opt for curtains that complement wall colors, preferably lighter shades. Cloth curtains provide a budget-friendly means to enhance the bathroom's appearance, and regularly changing clear liners keeps everything pristine.

5. Bathtub Caddy:

If indulging in baths is part of your self-care routine, a bathtub caddy becomes a valuable accessory. It keeps all your supplies – from bath salts and oils to cleansing soap and a good book – within easy reach, eliminating the need to disrupt your relaxation by getting out of the water.

6. Waterproof Bluetooth Speaker:

Elevate your bathroom experience from mundane to enjoyable by introducing a waterproof Bluetooth speaker. Whether you're immersed in a bath or rushing through your morning shower, this speaker allows you to listen to your preferred tunes, enhancing the overall ambiance of your self-care moments.

Embracing the Healing Power of Indoor Greenery

For a reminder on why engaging with nature constitutes a form of self-care, revisit the section on forest bathing. While the idea of spending time in nature sounds appealing, the reality is that the average person spends 93 percent of their time indoors, making a 2-hour forest bath, or finding an accessible forest, often impractical due to time constraints. If you find yourself among those with limited time, that's perfectly fine. You can still enjoy some of the benefits akin to a forest bath from the convenience of your home. This is possible because the phytoncides responsible for reducing blood pressure, alleviating stress, and enhancing the immune system are not exclusive to outdoor plants; every plant produces them.

The straightforward solution lies in acquiring houseplants. Incorporating a touch of nature into your living space is a simple yet effective way to instantly enliven the atmosphere, induce relaxation, and contribute to your overall well-being. Research indicates that tending to and interacting with houseplants yields a similar sense of tranquility and stress relief as spending time with outdoor greenery. Beyond their aesthetic appeal, houseplants actively purify indoor air and might even enhance cognitive function. On an energetic level, the presence of living entities in your home fosters positive energy, helping dissipate any frenetic energy brought in from outside.

The challenge lies in caring for these plants. Much like all living organisms, plants require fundamental elements to flourish, and although understanding their needs may initially pose a challenge, with practice and patience, anyone can successfully nurture them.

Plants Resilient to Neglect

You don't need an expert green thumb to maintain plants successfully. Some plants, such as the ones listed below, are exceptionally resilient, making them ideal companions for those with a tendency for neglectful care.

1. Succulents: These trendy plants, ubiquitous in flower shops and trendy homes, boast a captivating appearance without demanding much attention. Hailing from arid climates, they store water and flourish in bright, warm light.

2. Snake Plants (Mother-in-law's Tongue): Recognizable for their long, sword-like spikes, these plants thrive in various light conditions, making them suitable for spaces with limited natural light. They tolerate irregular watering and may need repotting if they grow too tall.

3. Pothos: Dramatic climbers perfect for hanging or cascading over bookshelves, pothos plants adapt well to different light conditions but require consistent watering. Large, speckled leaves indicate health, while brown leaves signal thirst.

4. Spider Plant: With long, spindly leaves cascading from

pots, spider plants add a touch of drama to any space. They are undemanding, thriving with minimal water and light. As they mature, they produce offshoots that can be repotted.

5. Cacti: Well-suited for forgetful waterers, cacti, akin to succulents, thrive in bright sunlight. Perfect for windowsills or balconies, cacti require minimal care and tend to flourish when left to their own devices.

6. Bamboo: Frequently found in offices and malls, bamboo is resilient in various conditions. Thriving in both bright and low light, bamboo requires minimal water and isn't affected by air quality, making it a versatile choice for work desks or dimly lit rooms.

7. Aloe: As succulents, aloe plants demand little water but prefer bright light. Placing a potted aloe on a kitchen windowsill ensures easy access. Beyond its low-maintenance nature, the sap within the leaves offers potent burn-healing and skin-moisturizing properties, making it a practical addition to any home.

Keeping Your Plants Thriving

Maintaining plants is simpler than it appears; they share basic needs with humans and require a dash of patience.

1. Watering: All plants, including robust ones like succulents and cacti, need water to survive. Regular watering, typically once a week, is crucial. Thoroughly soak the soil in a circular motion, stopping when water begins to drain from the pot. Yellow leaves signal overwatering, while brown leaves indicate the need for more water.

2. Light: Plants rely on light for photosynthesis, transforming chlorophyll into food. Even those labeled as thriving in "low

light" still require some light to live. Instruction cards provided with purchased plants guide you on their light preferences. Direct light suits windowsills, indirect light suits shelves, and low light accommodates darker rooms with windows.

3. Air: Similar to humans, plants need proper airflow. Avoid confining them in closed-off spaces lacking air circulation. Ensure well-ventilated rooms with open windows, fans, or consider placing them on an outdoor porch or balcony.

4. Temperature: Many plants are temperature-sensitive. Be cautious around vents and heaters that, although not always active, can harm plants. For example, a plant thriving on a radiator in summer might suffer when the heater operates in winter, potentially scorching and killing the plant.

5. Pot Size: The pot size significantly impacts houseplants. Optimal sizing prevents excessive strain or insufficient space for growth. Consult store staff for the best pot size when purchasing a plant. Always choose pots with drainage holes to prevent waterlogging, and consider using saucers to contain any excess water.

6. Soil: Select specialized soil for potted plants, as it contains nutrients tailored for container environments. Avoid using soil from outdoor locations, as bagged soil is typically sterilized, protecting plants from pests and germs that could compromise both their health and your home.

Candles

The typical self-care scenario often portrays a woman indulging in a bubble bath, holding a glass of wine, with soft music and candlelight creating a soothing ambiance. This image is so ingrained that it's challenging to envision a tranquil bath without it. Despite being predominantly depicted with women in movies or on TV, this stereotype has contributed significantly to the misconception that candles are exclusively feminine. In reality, candles are inherently cool and arguably quite masculine. After all, what's more effortlessly guy-friendly than igniting something? Candles have an unparalleled ability to promptly alter the atmosphere of a space. The flame itself induces a calming effect, the gentle flickering light denotes relaxation, and specific scents exert tangible effects on the brain. The influence of scented candles extends beyond perception, as they genuinely and measurably impact the body, making them a valuable and prevalent tool in aromatherapy.

How Aromatherapy Operates:

Aromatherapy is grounded in the notion that distinct fragrances trigger responses in your brain. Scientifically validated, the olfactory receptors in your nose establish direct connections to your brain. Utilizing brain mapping, researchers have identified that specific scents induce reactions in distinct areas of your brain. For example, lavender has been shown to influence your brain's theta waves, associated with relaxation and drowsiness. Inhaling other scents can result in varied effects such as increased energy, enhanced focus, or stress reduction. Scientific evidence also supports the close connection between scent and memory, elucidating why certain fragrances can evoke forgotten moments from your past.

Why Opt for Candles?

It's straightforward. The heat and essential oils in the candle's wax efficiently diffuse scents into the air, known as the "hot throw." This indicates how rapidly a space becomes saturated with fragrance. High-quality candles boast a strong hot throw, requiring minimal burn time to circulate the scent. Experimenting with scents for brain manipulation involves finding one you enjoy. Light it when alone and observe your response – do you feel relaxed or more focused? Understanding the emotional impact guides your use. Some candles even label moods or settings (e.g., "relax" or "fireplace"). Keep it simple, choose a candle you like, and use it regularly.

There's no wrong time for a candle. Whether meditating, prepping for sleep, or enhancing your home's ambiance, candles fit any occasion. They're perfect after chores or baths, signaling a clean space. No special occasion is needed, but having one lit when company arrives improves the atmosphere.

For Men:

Selecting candles is personal, but newcomers can explore scents like:
- Sandalwood: Smoky with subtle sweetness.
- Pine: A year-round Christmas tree scent, instantly cozy.
- Patchouli: Earthy and musky, often blended with botanicals.
- Palo Santo: Smoky and purifying with a touch of mystery.
- Neroli: A citrusy, subtle, energizing scent evoking summer.
- Vetiver: Sharp and green, reminiscent of spring's first day.
- Leather: Warm and cozy, perfect for cold winter months, often mixed with other comforting notes.

Candle Safety Tips for those Fearful of Fire

If the thought of lighting a candle makes you uneasy, follow these straightforward steps to ensure safe burning.

1. Trim the Wick Regularly:

Ensure the wick remains short to keep the flame low and minimize smoke. Use a trimmer or scissors to cut the wick after each use.

2. Choose an Open Setting:

Avoid burning candles near potentially flammable items like papers, books, plants, or clothes. Place them on open tables or counters.

3. Never Leave Unattended:

Despite candles being in containers, there's still a risk of spillage or tipping. Never leave a burning candle unattended or place it where visibility is a challenge.

4. Stay Awake While Burning:

If you light a candle for relaxation, avoid leaving it burning overnight. Let the scent work its magic but extinguish the candle before bedtime.

5. Use a Snuffer:

If worried about wax splatter while blowing out candles, opt for a candle snuffer. It aids in extinguishing candles without creating a mess.

Set the mood with Fragrance

Candles serve a purpose beyond enhancing your home's scent or masking unpleasant odors. Aromatherapy's potency lies in its capacity to influence your emotions and mood. Whether preparing for a date or welcoming guests, candles can transform the perceived ambiance for both you and others. Consider these examples:

1. Calm and Relaxed:

Create a serene, spa-like atmosphere with candles featuring ingredients like lavender and eucalyptus.

2. Clean and Bright:

Illuminate a fresh and clean environment by burning candles with citrus notes such as lemon, bergamot, or neroli.

3. Cozy and Welcoming:

Infuse wintery notes like cinnamon, wood, and leather to add a warm, inviting touch, providing a fireplace-like ambiance.

4. Casual and Breezy:

Incorporate herbal scents like vetiver, rosemary, and basil to evoke a relaxed, open feel, making even a windowless space seem airy and spacious.

5. Sexy and Mysterious:

Set a smoky, sensual tone using candles with exotic notes like frankincense, sandalwood, and palo santo, signaling a seductive atmosphere.

Crafting a Fragrance Narrative

Men use cologne for various reasons – to boost confidence, add a touch of allure, attract attention, or mask less pleasant odors. Typically, cologne is seen as the finishing touch to a grooming routine, akin to the cherry on a sundae. A well-placed spritz of cologne possesses the remarkable ability to alter one's mood and conceal a range of scents.

However, many men limit their fragrance experience to personal grooming, overlooking the broader impact of scents on their lives, especially within their homes. While the scent of one's home may not seem significant, it undoubtedly matters. Have you ever entered a house and immediately sensed an unpleasant odor? The experience of stepping into a space with an off-putting smell can be challenging to shake off, even if you eventually adapt to it. On the contrary, recall a moment when you entered a home with a delightful fragrance – it elicited a positive feeling. Wouldn't you prefer to be the one with a pleasantly scented home?

This book has extensively discussed the benefits of aromatherapy, and it holds true – scents can influence your mood and activate specific areas of your brain. The challenge arises when your home has an undesirable smell, akin to living in a space filled with unpleasant scents that you eventually become immune to. Considering the impact of scents on mood, residing in a place with consistently unpleasant smells can be a downer. You might not even notice it until you implement a few changes.

Moreover, pleasant scents not only welcome visitors but also foster positivity. They possess the ability to conceal various aspects, as evident when hastily cleaning your place before guests arrive. A home that emanates delightful fragrances makes it less likely for guests to notice any underlying cleanliness issues. This alone should be motivation enough to prioritize a pleasing home scent.

<u>Selecting Your Fragrance Arsenal</u>

In the quest for a well-scented and uplifting home, you have an array of tools at your disposal, and the choice ultimately hinges on personal preference.

1. Candles:
   Scented candles reign supreme in the realm of home fragrances. Refer back to the preceding section for insights into their efficacy and usage.

2. Incense:
   Despite associations with college town head shops and formal church services, incense should not be underestimated. It swiftly saturates a space with fragrance, sparking conversations

and infusing an air of mystery.

3. Diffusers:

Advocates of diffusers argue that they surpass candles in terms of safety and effectiveness. Some use natural reeds immersed in essential oils, while others utilize small flames or plug into wall outlets. Generally subtler, diffusers provide a constant, subtle background aroma, distinguishing themselves from the rapid diffusion of candle scents.

4. Room Sprays:

Analogous to cologne for your home, room sprays are applied into the air, leaving a lingering scent. Unlike wearable fragrance, room sprays feature lighter molecules that remain suspended in the air for an extended period without requiring warmth for sustained fragrance.

5. Linen Sprays:

Recognizable as a household name like Febreze, high-quality linen sprays offer a distinct advantage over typical odor eliminators. Infused with essential oils, these sprays not only refresh your linens but also introduce aromatherapy benefits. For example, a lavender spray on sheets promotes better sleep, while eucalyptus spray neutralizes odors on pet-frequented areas of furniture.

6. Drawer Sachets:

Placing scented sachets in dresser drawers and closets accomplishes more than just preserving the freshness of your clothes. It serves as a deterrent to pests like moths. Confined spaces tend to trap odors and moisture, which can lead to a musty smell in stored clothing. Scented sachets help maintain control over these issues.

Crafting Your Distinctive Fragrance

Much like selecting a cologne, curating the scent of your home demands careful consideration to leave a lasting, positive impression.

1. Contemplate the Desired Mood:
Apply the principles of aromatherapy to home scenting. Tailor your choices to evoke specific moods; for a serene ambiance, opt for notes like lavender, while energizing citrus scents convey freshness. Wood and smoke scents contribute to a warm and cozy setting.

2. Mix Different Products:
Encourage discovery by combining various products such as candles and incense. Place these items strategically in different rooms to maintain an element of surprise. Remember, more potent doesn't always equate to better.

3. Draw Inspiration from Nature:
Even if sweet or food-inspired scents aren't your preference, nature provides excellent inspiration. Scents derived from trees, plants, and other natural sources are well-suited for spacious environments like homes. Consider the invigorating aroma of a pine-scented candle as a substitute for the fragrance of a Christmas tree.

4. Incorporate Living Elements:

Enhance the potency of natural-scented candles and diffusers by introducing living elements. Fresh flowers or fragrant plants complement these scents, providing layers of realism that go beyond what a candle alone can achieve. Choose plants with notes resembling those in your chosen candle or diffuser.

5. Establish a Theme:

Rather than overwhelming your space with a myriad of scents, select a theme and build upon it. Opt for multiple products sharing a common note; for example, if you favor wood scents, choose candles featuring sandalwood and distribute them throughout various rooms to maintain harmony.

6. Maintain Cleanliness:

To ensure your carefully crafted scents shine, eliminate potential competing odors. Regularly dispose of trash, clear dirty dishes from the sink, and stow away laundry. A pristine environment allows your chosen fragrances to take center stage.

The End

Thanks a lot for getting to this point dear Friend, if there's any chapter you don't understand, just read it over again and let it sink in.

In case you enjoyed this book, tell me what you enjoyed the most in the review section on the sales page. I hope the information in these pages have helped you.